A Rhythm of my Choosing

A journal of personal reflections

during a year with breast cancer

GW00746076

Sue Percival

Anchorage Publications
Durham, DH1 5LR
www.anchorage-publications.co.uk

The rights of Susan E Percival to be identified as the author
of this work have been asserted in accordance with
sections 77 and 78 of the Copyright Designs & Patents Act 1988.

British Library Cataloguing in Publication Data:
A catalogue record for this book is available
from the British Library

ISBN 978-0-9550311-1-3

Printed in England by
BookPrintingUK, Peterborough

Whilst we are in the vacuum between the operation and the start of chemotherapy, it is already evident that our lives are being controlled by others.

We must both hand ourselves over to these, as yet, strangers and trust their skills. But it's like being manipulated, marionette-like, through a routine that everybody knows but us; a secret composition of intricate and terrible design; a chorus of nurses and a cohort of registrars that have danced this macabre dance before, but this is not a rhythm of our choosing.

AUTHOR'S NOTE

This book is based on the diary I have kept during the year my life was consumed by the need to survive.

I wrote it mainly to keep me sane; my way of coping when my world turned upside down. I also used parts of it to keep friends updated with my progress in my fight against breast cancer.

Throughout my life, I have compulsively 'written things out of me'; rejoicing at good things, and consigning the not-so-good things to the past.

My story is not a rant against our local National Health Service Hospital, although you could, at times, be forgiven for thinking so.

Nor is it one intended to frighten you, if you or someone close to you may unfortunately have to embark on the same venture.

Some of the things that have happened to me along the way have been unusual and exceptional, well beyond the norm that one might expect.

If you, or someone you know, are facing this same illness, please remember the one mantra that has been repeated to me constantly by the professionals: *'Everyone is Different'*. I hope your loved one or friend will not experience too many of the problems and extremes that I encountered. Notwithstanding those, I survived against the odds.

This is simply **my** story, one of positivity and hope, against those odds, many of which were, sadly, man-made and unnecessary. I thank you for allowing me to share it with you.

My story is also one of thanksgiving, to those who have loved and supported me throughout the past year.

I am fortunate to have what people call a 'sunny personality'. I hope a little of the sunshine rubs off on you!

Sue Percival

June 2009

CONTENTS

Dedication

This book is lovingly dedicated to my amazing husband without whom I
simply would not have survived.

Appreciation:

*To all who have encouraged me to record this unwanted journey, and to
Aaron Carr (artwork); Steve Rooke (editing); Mike Amos (foreword);
Cass Nightingale (medical)*

FOREWORD

Most of us have our "hospital" stories. I remember while in coronary care – false alarm, good intent – learning that "Mint imperial" was rhyming slang for "immaterial".

I remember being wheeled into A&E whilst wearing one black shoe and one brown one – at least they were *otherwise* identical – and I remember, in the middle of the dark night of the sole room occupant, being absurdly cheered by the insistence of the bed-end chart that my height-to-weight index was normal.

That was while being treated for a deep vein thrombosis, what the medics call a DVT. Even a DVT might be preferable to a PFI, but that's another story. It's Sue Percival's, and it's utterly compelling.

There's been a rash (to maintain a vaguely medical metaphor) of medical "diaries", usually concerning a battle with cancer. Hitherto the most memorable, certainly the most saturnine in its humour, was written by Dominic Lawson, every Saturday in The Times.

Maybe I thought Sue's account was going to be similar to most of the others: courageous, honest but a little self-serving. Maybe - for I'm so cowardly, I could be an exhibit in the Squeamish Museum - I wondered why Sue and Allan had asked me to write the foreword. Maybe I thought, after the diagnosis of that lump beneath her arm on April 1st 2008, that it would be just another case of duck egg blues.

What a fearful misdiagnosis. Sue's account is much more uncomfortable than that.

While necessarily it chronicles her personal battle for survival, the awful awareness that just when nothing else can possibly go wrong it usually does, it has another and yet more dreadful element.

It tells of the systemic failings of the health service and, in particular, of one "flagship" Private Finance Initiative NHS hospital – not the best place to be, as at one desperate stage she concludes, but the worst.

"How can I possibly trust my life to this hospital?" she asks at one agonised stage. I'd have named the place but Sue – doubtless wisely, for she's had enough problems of late – chooses not to.

No sub-plot is needed, but one arrives in her elderly mother-in-law's illness, and in the awful, familiar, awfully familiar nightmares that are its bedfellows: the absence of dignity or of basic hygiene, the shortage of staff, the failure to understand even the most basic protocols. Then there's the new doctor who insists they've been taught how to deal with patients who are hard of hearing and proceeds to bellow in her ear.

Is anybody listening?

Incorrigibly, indelibly, I tend to mark books for review with felt tip pen, emphasising those passages to which I might want to return. Like a bed-end chart in an intensive care unit, the marks on Sue's text became ever more frequent. This is becoming worrying; this is serious; this may be a national emergency.

Is there still nobody listening; listening to the patient?

It's flattering to be asked by one whose own love of language is so manifest to contribute a foreword. In the email to which the text was attached, however, Allan hoped that there'd also be a comment from a prominent medical consultant. That, goodness knows, should be the really interesting addition. Something from the Department of Health – some hope – might have been better yet.

Inevitably, there are reasons to be cheerful, chiefly in Sue's indomitable (most of the time) spirit, in the abiding love of Allan, of family and friends – best include the dog in that, too – and in the excellence of the new Northern Centre for Cancer Care, in Newcastle.

Best of all, of course, is that she lives to tell the tale in a way that is at times as brutal as it is careful, but always beautifully and thoughtfully crafted. We must all thank God for that.

Mike Amos MBE
The Northern Echo

Chapter 1

A HEALTH WARNING FOR THE READER!

Why?

It is not the question "Why me?"

There is little point in wasting emotion on such a question.
Breast cancer is all around me. Several friends have suffered it, and survived it, before it became my turn. In fact, at times, it seems like an epidemic.

The question "Why?" is behind my reasoning for wanting to publish this little book. In wanting to see this story in print, I have had to ask myself 'why'; to question my motives.

After all, it is in the major part, pretty harrowing, hence a health warning! The reason has nothing to do with ego. I have written more than enough poetry, which has been enjoyed by so many people.

It is very likely that I would not have chosen to read a book such as this just as I was embarking on this unwanted trip of a lifetime. I found it difficult enough to read the Cancer support websites at times, as too much information all at once can be difficult to cope with. Others may disagree.

I would like to think this book would be read by health professionals involved in cancer care, strategic planning and hospital organisation, management and staff training. Hopefully it would benefit their understanding of what it is like from the patient's side of the mountain.

But it is so much more than that. I have already said my story is not the common experience for most people who have made this same journey. In some ways, I was unlucky; in others, very fortunate. Many people are able to carry on working through chemotherapy and lead reasonably normal lives. Others have rough passages on the way. Mine was more difficult than that. As with others before me, I happened to be given a particularly hard route to survival.

Part of the reason behind my wanting this story read is as a salute to those who saw me through it; who loved me through it. Another is to demonstrate how we all need to question everything and not blindly accept what we are told, and what is being done to us.

And finally, it is about surviving the best way we can; learning to ask for the right kind of help, and accepting all the help that is thrown at us.

A close friend who lived it through with me, and read the draft of this story before I decided to publish, said of it,

"In all its glory, as you describe your harrowing death defying journey, your sunny nature wins through. As I read, I felt uplifted as time and again you demonstrated strengths of spirit that are truly amazing, humbling and awe inspiring.

By the end, I did not feel miserable. I was joyful that I still have the pleasure and privilege of having you in my life".

In quoting this, I do not wish to demonstrate my own qualities, whatever they are, but to say again and again, I did not do this alone. I would not have been strong enough. It was a communal effort, for which I am entirely in other people's debt. In retrospect, as I read this through now, it seems that I was trapped in a time capsule; one of horror and fear which now seems so alien to my personality. But none of us knows how we will react to different circumstances which are beyond our experience and understanding.

I really am not a very demanding person. I have not demanded much of my life, although it would seem I have achieved all I could wish for......to date! I don't demand too much of others either. I am lucky enough to be able to accept them as they are, and if knowing each other can brighten both our lives a little, I am happy. The only important thing in life, in my view, is to be happy, and to make others around you happy. Nothing else matters.

My passions are really simple. I love words, and I love writing them, and encouraging others to enjoy them too. And I enjoy people. Behind every face is a story. We may bemoan our lot, but others always have a story to tell too. The poetry within this book is part of my coping and survival process. I wrote it as I travelled along this unwanted route.

But for one moment in time, all this was beyond me. I could only bury myself in a dark place and hide. Once surgery was decided upon, I could do no more. Not for one moment did it frighten me. My fears were now behind me, from the very point of diagnosis. The truly terrifying part was in not knowing my enemy. I approached surgery without any fear at all. My fear was simply of my promised future.

9

THE GARDEN

A garden was planted,
and around her feet
lovely flowers sprang;
unheard of flowers
of a strange beauty
and mystery,
until that moment never seen before.

People came to see
the wondrous sight,
entranced by the
child-like pleasure
that was taken
by one who had
until that moment never known before.

And they plucked
the flowers
which she gladly gave,
each bloom a little
different from the last;
fragrant perfumes
until that moment never smelt before.

But she didn't know
that in the bouquet
of beautiful blooms
was a stem with a thorn
which was plucked
and pricked those who
until that moment had never been hurt before.

Author's Note
*As you read through this book you will notice entries in italics;
these words were written after each episode, as a reflection.*

Chapter 2

SURVIVAL – a NEW CHAPTER

11th April

Nothing in my eventful life has prepared me for this latest chapter. The last two weeks, since Easter Monday when I found a 'duck egg' had been laid under my arm overnight, have been the most horrifying to endure, forcing me into a nightmare world within myself. I try to share it, but most of it is locked inside where it is impossible for others to reach.

And yet, strangely, the fear is mostly of the effect on those around me, and I bargain with the gods that this will be just my mountain to climb.

I disintegrate and curl up in a ball on the settee, weepingly retreating into myself. Part of me is ashamed of my lack of coping, while the other parts are obliterated by fear.

I am very aware of the need to immediately address the phenomenon. I know that time is of the essence.

The following day I am given an urgent appointment to see my GP, who examines me both then and four days later, to see if there is any change.

Easter Monday was actually our Wedding Anniversary, but we were to find ourselves consumed in very different depths of love on this significant day; one borne of understanding, sharing and supporting each other through many wonderful years of marriage.

We shared tears that evening, and a closeness that gave each of us strength. But we both knew that it would be me who had to face the toughest of physical and mental challenges as this story unfolded.

We have been with our General Practice since first moving to the outskirts of Durham City some thirty five years ago. There have been very few problems in this relationship and we have respected their professionalism.

Having trained as a nurse when I left school and then become a Staff Nurse until a back injury removed me from the profession, I have an instinctive medical understanding. Our daughter has inherited that trait, using her skills to study in palaeopathology. Between us, we can usually make an educated guess at many ailments.

I had not missed the arrival of this duck-egg, although there must have been some invisible signs.

It appeared overnight, giving no warning, and no time for observation and interpretation, but we were all quietly aware of the possibility of its origin and likely sinister intent.

We had now embarked on an unwanted but very welcome newfound understanding with all members of the Practice team, from receptionists through to GPs. From the outset, one of us had simply to contact them with a concern or a request for medications and they proved instantly supportive.

This support helped to make our lives so much easier. They have continued such support to this day.

I decide I cannot wait for an NHS appointment, even the fast track route for potential cancer sufferers. Instead, we arrange to see a Consultant urgently, via the private route. I feel instinctively that the delay has been too long already, although it is only a week since the lump appeared.

I am given the first available appointment; it will be in the evening of April Fools' Day.

I attend a nearby private hospital, where I sit in terror, waiting for my name to be called. I cannot believe it is really me sitting there. The waiting room is full of people who look normal and carefree-but maybe some of them who are suffering like me are simply good at hiding their fear.

When I am examined, the Consultant can tell there is a lump in my breast as well as the highly obvious one under my arm.

Suddenly, so swiftly, I find myself on a nightmare conveyer belt. Mammogram is followed by an ultrasound scan, and then by many needle biopsies. It is all outside my control, and I shake so much on the table, a Sister holds me down to keep me still. No matter what I had been preparing myself for, I am in physical shock. Each biopsy taken seems to the surgeon to be normal in appearance. He takes more and more, which, he says, is an uncommon thing to have to do. And my fear grows.

My breast is bruised and battered from the many biopsies, but deep inside me, I already know it doesn't matter. I know the breast will not be there at all for much longer.

≈≈≈≈≈

The diagnosis, a few days later, is a relief. After two weeks of what has seemed an endless endurance trial, I now know what my battle will be, and who my enemy is.

Grade Three aggressive cancer cells have been found under my arm, but the many biopsies taken from my breast are found to be benign. Yet the surgeon is convinced the same cancer will be in my breast somewhere. Why else would it be found under my arm?

We discuss the options, although in reality there are none. Surgery will be followed by chemotherapy, and then radiotherapy. My surgeon tells me that the six months of chemotherapy will soon pass! But first, we must consider the route surgery will take. At my first appointment, I had hoped my breast could be saved. Now, knowing what I may have, I just want the evil parasite taken from my body as soon as possible.

I have a choice: take a gamble and just have a surgical biopsy to prove it is there, and thereby risk a delay which may be dangerous. Or take a gamble and have a mastectomy, relying on the surgeon's intuition. In truth, there is no choice.

My fight begins from that moment. And I can fight. I feel so strong. My husband Allan and I make the decision to tell our family and friends everything, from the outset. We will all need support.

Our daughter is immediately pragmatic and seeks to ease our fears by research and logic. Allan's elderly Mum had been through a similar scare twenty-five years earlier. Living alone, she has much time to "think" and to dwell upon this news. She is so supportive, but she also needs much support from us. Our son and daughter- in- law are on holiday and we decide to wait for their return before breaking the news.

There can never be an easy way to share such news and when we meet them, it is evident by our demeanour that bad news is coming. Naturally, their immediate reaction is of shock and concern, instantly followed by assurances that whilst they might not be able to contribute to "medical" needs, they would do everything practical.

My whole family's strength and support is to prove invaluable over the following months.

The resultant outpouring of love from all the walks of my life astounds me. It is a living eulogy, and I am so privileged to know how much I am loved; how much we as a family are loved and supported. I feel humbled.

There is no decision to be made. Surgery is inevitable and I know it must be radical. I don't face it alone. I am never alone. The love that surrounds me takes this journey with me.

Thanks to a caring, intuitive surgeon, who has led me gently to this decision, I feel safe and confident. In his hands, I know I have the best chance possible with a total mastectomy, and I do not hesitate. The test results have indicated there can be no further delay and the surgeon's prognosis is that *any* delay will prove detrimental.

We immediately agree not to wait for the NHS route, regardless of how many times I am told by outsiders there will be no delay (*subsequently we would learn this was a complete fallacy)* but decide instead to take the private path, even though we do not have insurance to cover the cost.

The much heralded new NHS Choose & Book scheme was just being launched in this very month of April. A lengthy phone conversation with the C&B Helpdesk confirmed that even on the day of my operation our choice of using a private, NHS approved, hospital was acceptable. In fact, this proved too soon for the local County NHS Trust to have policies, practices and understanding in place for me to use this route. And our debate about that failure and interpretation by the Trust continues at the time of writing these words, one year later.

A few days - and several further tests later, I enter my chosen Private Hospital and I am very fortunate to be in a place where I am so well cared for. I have no fears. I place myself entirely in their hands and no longer have to concern myself with the battle.

The love I feel here too, is humbling; from my gentle welcome at admission, on to walking down the corridor to the Operating Theatre with Allan, where he kisses me at the door, and places me in the care of the competent, kind anaesthetic staff.

Immediately post-surgery, the surgeon further confirms that another two weeks of living with this traitor would have meant a very different ending to this chapter and my life expectancy. Just two weeks.

Twenty-four hours after surgery I am up, exercising for the first time in the corridor outside my room – three double lengths, carrying my drain bottles in my hand. I am met by a Staff Nurse who hugs me, kisses me on the cheek, and says, 'Look at you! You're a star!'

And I feel it! It is another blessing in my life.

The sense of loss, when it comes, is palpable. But it is not the loss of a breast, but the destruction of the traitor lurking inside me. I feel no forfeiture of 'womanhood'.

Once again, I count my blessings. I know there are difficult days ahead. I know I will feel very differently at times. But for the present, I count those blessings and deal with *now*.

I seem to be filled with energy. I think I am resting, although I am not sleeping. It is 3am as I write this. I have slept, but woken, and am pampered with hot milk and toast! Instead of the noise and chaos of previous hospital experiences, I am cosseted! It is so peaceful here and I feel so safe. Again, and again, I count my blessings.

Within the space of only twenty-four hours I am off oxygen, detached from the monitor, my drip is down, and the calf pulsators removed. I regain my independence and freedom. Only the drains to go now, but even with them I am able to feel normal again. The pain is really quite insignificant today. I just have to move carefully, and especially remember the drainage bottles! I put them down, and when I pick them up I talk to them saying 'come on dogs, we're going for a walk.' Better that than forgetting them and walking off without them! That would really hurt!

I am allowed to take a shower, and wash my hair. Alone, I strip naked, negotiating drainage tubes and emotions. In the mirror, I look at my plastic-covered lopsided chest, but feel only relief. I can cope with this. All that matters is that I am the victor.

12th April

This morning I have had a chance to catch up on my book of daily poetry readings. So I start with April 10th, surgery day. I am delighted to see it is Keats':

A thing of beauty is a joy forever

Its loveliness increases, it will never

Pass into nothingness, but still keep

A bower quiet for us, and a sleep

Full of sweet dreams, and health and quiet breathing.

Therefore, on every morrow, we are wreathing

A flowery band to bind us to the earth

'Spite of despondence.

I can think of no better words to guide me on my new 'adventure'.

≈≈≈≈≈

But the day descends into a difficult one. I cannot stop weeping.
Those around me, caring for me, know, and are always on hand if I need them.

As always, I write it out of me:

16

THE OTHER HALF

The other half of me

sneaks out

and attacks me while my guard is down.

Unexpectedly

it weaves its way around me,

surrounding me with anguish,

and will not let me go.

I close every pore to it

retreating to my hidden self,

denying access of my core to it.

The better half of me

waits by

to sustain and hold me, guide me

supportingly,

and weaves its way around me,

surrounding me with love.

I will not let it go.

14th April

My emotions swing; euphoria sometimes, knowing how near to the edge I've come. At the other end of the scale, not despair, just the fear of what I have to face in the near future. I shake those feelings off, and close that door; time enough to open it. For now, I content myself with my present battle. Strangely, it feels already won. I have faced the worst for the time being, and come through with honours. Thanks to the fortune of good timing, wise counsel and prompt action.

None of this is easy; not for me, nor for those who love me. But we all have a purpose, together. I have never drifted along in my life. I have embraced it with enthusiasm, and that hasn't changed. Life has always had so much meaning for me, maybe simply because it has never been easy. But I climb these new 'Meetings with Fate' – enormous mountains mostly – and find that the view from the summit is one of open skies and sunlight. It is never dark on a mountain top, so the climb is never in vain.

15th April

Sandy, our lovely dog, has many toys, and they are all named. He is clever enough to identify and favour many of them. So far, he can identify more than a dozen by name, and the list - and his skill -continues to grow.

One of them is a small bow shape, made of soft material with a squeak in the middle. He treats it so gently, and never hurts it, just makes it squeak. It is called Softie.

I knew that getting dressed to go home would be hard. It would be the first time the change in me would be obvious, not just to me but also to others. I had packed the right underwear and had mentally prepared myself for it, as I had prepared myself for the first look in the mirror on my first day out of bed.

At the hospital, when I had dressed to go home, I went and had a word with the Sister.

I said,
'When I get home all the family will be there, and, people being human, their eyes are bound to go straight to the spot. Tell me honestly, is this absence a bit too obvious for them to cope with?'

She said,

'Sue, I've the very thing for you, it just tapes to the inside of your clothes, and no-one will tell. It's filled with a soft fibre so you can adjust the size to match. Come into my room and we'll sort you out. It's called a Softie'. Sorry to disappoint............... it doesn't squeak!

But my dearest friend this morning assured me I may find a tassel for it!

Interestingly, Sandy had never been allowed into our bedrooms but after my return home from hospital he knew that I was home and pined dreadfully to see me and be near me. The decision was therefore reached (with him having the casting vote!) that he would be allowed into my bedroom so that he could see me.

Of course, he had other plans! Having entered the room, in one bound he was onto the bed and, just as quickly, had snuggled himself alongside me – thankfully on my"good" side and without causing me any pain.

Over the weeks and the months I was confined to bed, Sandy would be my constant carer. When I was able to rest or sleep downstairs during daytimes, he would be curled on the floor immediately beside me. There was never any argument that during the night, he would sleep in his usual place downstairs, but in the mornings, immediately he had been into the garden and had his breakfast, he had one key responsibility – looking after me.

He knew, before even I did, when I was going to cry. He would nuzzle his head into my neck, bringing solace and comfort BUT he also knew when I was going to be sick – and he'd be down the stairs and hiding under Allan's desk before I'd even reached for the vomit bowl!

ANTICIPATION

I watch the clock
having watched the calendar
for so long.

No longer counting days
I count the hours,
heartbeats converted into seconds,
seconds into dreams.

I watch and wait,
seeing things in slow motion,
hearing sounds through an
old phonograph, winding down,
making idiotic sense.

I am impatient,
willing time to fly
that I might flee.
And yet when my time comes
I will command the clock to cease
as kings once commanded the sea.

Chapter 3

AND IT'S ONLY JUST BEGINNING

19TH April

It is nine days post-surgery, and in the scheme of things, I'm doing really well. Only nine days.

I have had my post-op outpatient meeting with the surgeon, something I was dreading. I had heard all the bad news, hadn't I? Yet still I dreaded the very thought of walking into the hospital where the first consultation was given - walking once again, through those doors; sitting in the busy waiting room and waiting to be called. It filled me with fear just to think about it. I'm glad I didn't have the surgery in that particular bustling private hospital, but had chosen another.

When the day finally arrived, I was strangely calm. The panic receded. Surely, I had already heard the worst. Absorbed it, coped with it, and swiftly dealt with it.

The wound is healing well, although the pain has increased quite a bit. But in my strange little way, I am pleased about that since it means that life is returning to it, and the peripheral nerves are doing their job, taking over from the severed ones.

We are finally informed of the histology results. The surgeon is completely sure that the entire tumour was excised, and none had adhered to any of the surrounding tissue. It had been hiding under a benign tumour – which explained all those negative biopsies- and had grown to twenty-two millimetres. In a very short space of time, fifteen of my eighteen axillary lymph nodes had all been invaded, and this aggressive grade three cancer was in all fifteen. But all have been cleanly removed along with the unaffected chest and neck nodes.

I am filled with horror that it could have been so swift and aggressive, but so very grateful for the surgeon's confidence and skill. Even more horrifying is that if we had followed the NHS route it would have been too late. No doubt about it. £3,760 (including VAT!!) well spent.

Immediately post-operation, the surgeon had told Allan that another ten to fourteen days would have been too late. He reminded us again of this harsh fact: if I had been diagnosed in the one-stop-breast clinic at our local NHS 'flagship, state of the art' hospital it would, he explained, have taken more than three weeks for surgery, therefore a possible total delay of over five weeks.

He already had six cancer patients waiting for urgent surgery (some breast, some neck/thyroid) and he cannot get the theatre space at the hospital to operate on those people any earlier, regardless of the urgency. He is only allocated one and a half theatre days a week (nothing to do with his private commitments - that is all the hospital can allow him). One of his theatre days is a Monday, and if that falls on a Bank holiday, he loses that week, and the patients wait a week longer. We are into the April/May Bank Holiday season and it is evidently clear I would not have survived. I count my blessings yet again.

An early appointment is to be confirmed with the Oncologist now. This is my next mountain. I am to be handed over to that department. It is in the local NHS hospital, but at least I will only be an out-patient, and I will have more control. *(Oh, how naive that seems with hindsight!)* I now have to face the challenge of chemotherapy and radiotherapy. The promised plans of spring-time and the summer dissolve before my eyes.

My emotions still swing like a pendulum. I do remain positive – that is never in question. With the prayers of Hindu, Muslim, Hebrew, Witness and Christian friends rooting for me I have no choice! Those, plus another friend's distance Reiki healing, cover all the bases and whether I believe or not, I embrace them all!

Cards and flowers continue to arrive daily. So many messages of love and support sustain us all. Our grown-up children show us both such maturity and love. And all around, the house is festooned with the cards and poems from the school children who give me such joy when I am sharing with them my love of the English language.

Yet I find myself suddenly quietly weeping at my loss. Not the loss of a breast – never that – but the loss of my freedom, my carefree days. Susie seems to be misplaced, leaving behind just me in this velvet prison. I resent my loss of energy, my drive. And I fear the months ahead – not the outcome, I have total confidence – but the changes they will force upon me. But I know Susie is still there inside me, waiting.

LITTLE GIRL LOST

Not lost
but hiding.
Not gone
but waiting.
Her time will come again.

Her smile still there,
the light in her eyes;
her joy of life
and gratitude for love.

Not lost
but hiding.
Her time is now
and always will be.

Little girl found.

FLUTTERING

A window opens
and an opportunity flies in
for me to grasp,
to hold.

Like a moth fluttering in my hand

But a moth will beat its wings
within my touch,
attracted by the light
in desperation to be free.

Such futility,
since freedom cannot be
so bravely sought
by man or moth, but given.

Like a cord severed in my soul

And so the moth might beat its way
within my touch,
attracted by my light
in anticipation, to be free

Until the window closes once again

Chapter 4

SKIN DEEP

28th April

And the next phase begins. I have met with the Oncologist, an up-front, head-on, type of woman; right up my street. Now I know what I have to face next, what *we* have to face next, since I don't embark on this alone, and I am so grateful for that. My heart goes out to the people who have tackled this nightmare without the support that I am so fortunate to have.

We discuss side effects of chemotherapy, and I have to sign a consent form, not only to have the treatment, but also to say I understand the possibility of certain side effects which have been explained to me. They include hair loss, increased risk of infection, nausea, tiredness, poor appetite, nail changes, and a possibility of an allergic reaction to one particular drug that will be used. This list includes definite ones and possible ones. It is intended to cover all eventualities.

But they do not include some that I will eventually have to suffer. Little do I know at this stage that I shall have every one of those in the book, and more beside!

Allan is quick to advise the Oncologist that I tend to be an awkward customer! I already have enough food allergies and drug sensitivities to cope with each normal lifestyle day, and he ensures that she is made aware of these. We ask our questions, and get straight-forward answers which I appreciate. Of course, I've been reading up on it all, as much as I can. I ask about using a cold cap to protect me from hair loss. Back comes the answer: why protect a single cell in my body, when I am going to have chemotherapy to reduce the slightest possible risk of the disease spreading? I decide bald is best!

I have to face a barrage of tests. They themselves are painless, but the fear behind them is awful. They are to check if this enemy has invaded any other part of me. The chemotherapy will start on May 14th, with an orientation in the Unit two days previously. I know that mountain will be a difficult one, but my fear of further invasion is worse, and I will be glad to get these tests over.

My days are fairly positive and confident, but my mood swings to the dark side in the evenings when I am tired. The panic descends on me then and is beyond my control. I discover that I don't have courage. The tears assault me and I cannot cope with them. I feel so sorry for Allan who suffers because I am beyond help when I get like this.

I have been advised by a friend to create a chart and mark each milestone as I pass it. We decide not on a cross or tick, but a gold heart as a sign of positivity! I must learn to treat these tests as positive things, and the chemotherapy treatment as an army of friendly soldiers.

I wonder about the wig. I hate hats and scarves, and I know I won't be very comfortable, but no doubt, pride will overcome that. I am fortunate to see a notice on the wall in the out-patients' waiting area. It tells me there is a charity called Headstrong, and as soon as I am able to, we go there. It is located in a Tyneside Hospice, which I find a little disconcerting, but I soon discover that Hospices have more than one purpose. Two volunteers, themselves survivors, give me advice beyond measure, and teach me how to tie headscarves in various ways. I am able to buy a selection of scarves and hats from them, very cheaply. I even buy a false fringe which can be stuck on the inside of the scarf, and I get a 'sleeping hat' too, as they tell me it can be quite draughty at night with no hair!

I feel I learn more in an hour from these women, than from all the health professionals put together! We learn from each other's mistakes and experience with such as:

> how vulnerable our skin is after chemotherapy;

> the importance of sun protection, forever;

> keeping up the arm exercises, long after radiotherapy is over;

> taking care of the mastectomy arm, protecting it from zealous nurses who try to use a blood pressure monitor on it, and from those who try to take blood from it;

> which shampoos to use – and when eventually returning to a hairdresser, taking my own shampoo and baby's brush with me

> always wearing gloves for gardening;

> avoiding cat litter.

I gain a myriad of useful advice which will stay with me forever, along with the kindness of those ladies who willingly give up their time for me and for others.

We later visit a hidden away, 1st floor, Gateshead shop named "Bouncing Back" which is run by a survivor and her mother. Again, their kindness and practical advice in finding suitable underwear is invaluable. I am measured without embarrassment. She has been there before me and whilst she can talk to me about her experience as a survivor, her Mum talks to Allan as one who became a carer! It is all a completely new learning experience.

Whilst we are in the vacuum between the operation and the start of chemotherapy, it is already evident that our lives are being controlled by others. We must both hand ourselves over to these, as yet, strangers and trust their skills. But it's like being manipulated, marionette-like, through a routine that everybody knows but us; a secret composition of intricate and terrible design; a chorus of nurses and a cohort of registrars that have danced this macabre dance before, but this is not a rhythm of our choosing. The routine may briefly slow but we can never rest, no matter how much we want to; each step another shift in the tempo of treatment, each treatment a recovery-related rhyme of sometimes interminable complexity.

I have been given plenty to read about side effects. And I am assured by the Oncologist that this chemical army will take care of any enemy that may have strayed, but still I panic in the dark hours, curled up inside myself, in a tight ball. This is a hard road to walk.

4th May

The worst is over! I have climbed the mountain, and the view from the summit is wonderful after all. I feel that I've been given my life back. All tests are negative; bones, abdomen, and lungs are all unaffected. The enemy has not spread. After a frightening false reading, my heart is apparently found to be capable of withstanding the chemotherapy. Some tests are conducted in the Nuclear Medicine department. Scary stuff! I am injected with radio-active dye, and am only allowed to pee in a special toilet! The machinery is enormous and fascinating.

As I lie there, I gaze at the paintings on the ceiling, placed there to amuse and calm children. It is a sobering thought to consider these children. But my tests are over, and I can briefly relax again. The relief is indescribable. There are simply no words available for this wordy person to use!! Now it is onwards and upwards!

SKIN DEEP

Where did she go,
lost in the poetic mists of time,
left incomplete,
no longer finished?
Where did she lose herself?

Words echo in her head
and time loses meaning.
Confusion builds
and weariness engulfs.
Where did she go?

Reflections puzzle
and confuse her,
driving her
to hidden depths.
Where did she go?

Changed beyond her control
But wait!

It is only skin deep.

14th May

I enter the Chemotherapy Unit of the hospital, having had my orientation a couple of days earlier. I am not fearless, but I'm not frightened, since this is inevitable, and I cannot avoid it. It is actually called 'Medical Investigations Unit' on the sign outside, with Chemotherapy written small, as if an afterthought. Perhaps 'Chemotherapy' is not an acceptable term to display in large letters to the public.

The orientation was conducted by a very caring, practical and professional Staff Nurse. She exuded so much confidence and positivity – and that was something I dearly needed. Allan accompanied me, to ensure no instructions or guidelines were forgotten and we both felt that most of our concerns had been addressed.

It was at this meeting we learnt about the **two-hour ruling** *– a rule that would come to haunt us over the coming weeks and months.* It was:

If my temperature should rise and remain above a minimum of
thirty-eight degrees for one hour, we must contact the Unit or
The Haematology ward. The seriousness was explained in great detail –
no deviation from that rule was permitted, for we were told repeatedly,
early death could be the outcome of ignoring it.
We were made very aware that time was of the essence.

Among other things, chemotherapy reduces the white cell count drastically, thereby reducing the body's ability to defend itself against infection, however minor.

I was issued with my dreaded "red book", the passport I would carry with me to every medical encounter over the next nine months. It provided not only my identity within "the system" but also my new medications, emergency contact numbers, and general information, plus further emphasis about the two hour rule. At first, this little red book was of strength to me, but I came to loathe it. The very sight of it would make me feel nauseous.

In fact, the very word 'chemotherapy' would make me nauseous!

Perhaps we should have been more "aware" at that meeting; perhaps we should, even then, have recognised the warning lights that flashed for us; perhaps we were carried along by the professionalism of the Staff Nurse and accepted all that took place. We had already acknowledged we had joined a moving conveyor belt from which there could be no stepping off, being carried along it in fulfilment of established treatment regimes on an odyssey over which we had no control.

We are told that an extra treatment day for breast cancer patients has recently been introduced, in response to increased demand, and this has eased some of the strain on the department.

Towards the end of that meeting, I was asked if I had any concerns or questions – and I had many! Sadly the conveyor belt had already failed me, for I had not been assigned a Breast Care Nurse; a point the Unit Sister would subsequently pursue on my behalf. A patient would normally be able to contact their designated Breast Care Nurse to discuss any concerns, but I (at that stage) knew no different and had struggled along.

Of greatest concern was that the area around my operation site was both very inflamed and full of fluid that could not drain. The Staff Nurse was concerned enough to decide I must be seen by a doctor immediately, who would then decide whether I should commence chemotherapy two days hence.

In our ignorance and innocence, we expected to be seen by an Oncologist, or a breast cancer specialist who, surely, formed part of the Unit staff. In the event, I was seen by one of the general surgical team of doctors on call within the hospital. He was very reassuring and felt there was no infection, but this was not his field of expertise and he could not advise whether I should commence treatment or not.

I recalled that my surgeon had told me that if ever I had a post-operative problem I should contact him and, indeed, I had seen him three times since the operation for him to aspirate the wound with a needle and syringe. I mentioned this to the staff and they agreed to ask whether he was in the hospital. Thankfully, for me, he was, and within twenty minutes, we were on his ward and he was examining me. He decided I should commence chemotherapy as planned.

Incidentally, this was a Monday. We were later to discover, as I lay at death's door in that hospital a few weeks later, a visiting Oncologist is only present on a Wednesday, when an outpatient clinic is held.

COURAGE

And so it begins;
a new mountain to climb,
new territory to explore.
A barren landscape
yet to be planted
with feelings, and later
long distant memories
which will fade.

I will paint this landscape
with the colour of hope,
and it will be bathed in
the sunlight of love.
And over it all
will be a rainbow of courage

(written on my first day of chemotherapy)

Treatment

The Unit is well designed with a couple of desks at the door, so you don't have to search around for help as you arrive. A member of staff is always there to welcome you. There is a comfortable looking waiting area, with armchairs, a coffee table, with books and information, and a bowl of chocolates. (I am to learn later that many people can never look at these kinds of chocolates again as they bring back too many awful memories). But for now, I am in total ignorance, and luckily for me, I am allergic to chocolate anyway!

On one side of this waiting area is a curtained- off room where treatment is given to people sitting in chairs, and at the other end, beds for those less able to sit. In between is a private interview room, and in the corridor a trolley where we can help ourselves to tea and coffee.

But I am to discover that it would seem the architects of this hospital didn't take volume of patients into consideration. The 'restful' waiting area is used as an overspill. There is very little room for relatives, should you feel the need for company, and no privacy at all. Patients with drips in their arms occupy most of the seats; some with chemotherapy dripping through, others with blood transfusions. I become used to the sight and sounds of pumps, constantly beeping and patients with bowls of hot water on lap pillows, with arms dangling to encourage reluctant veins.

I suppose in a way I am fortunate. I go to the cubicle area since my chemotherapy involves several large syringe-full's being slowly pushed into my canular which is inserted (with increasing difficulty) every time I go. To do this, a Sister has to sit opposite me and it is done over a long period of time. Each syringe has its own little quirky way with me! One makes my bottom itch terribly for a few seconds; another immediately makes my nose run, and another makes my urine red for a few days. It is all so alien to start with, but becomes familiar very quickly.

The nurses are kind, but so very busy. There are so many of us patients. We meet each other and we share our stories; some needing to talk about their condition. It is a little like a club to which you would much rather not belong and some stories you would prefer not to hear. I try to retreat into myself, cut myself off, and write it out of me.

And so my nightmare begins.

WEAKNESS

First numb and silent,
her mind now will not let her be.
Her body betrays her with its weakness
and her heart gives up its secrets.
Words stumble their way
over the rocks and canyons
until they bleed through every pore.
They will not give her peace.

She writes them down, but still
they will not leave her.
She tries to occupy her thoughts
with mundane things,
but energy is sapped and drained
and offers no support
in resisting and repelling.

The force is beyond control.
Far stronger
than the frail and timid body.
Far more determined
than the weak and futile mind.

Such words.
Braver than she.

During this time, I am at last assigned a Breast Care Nurse. She has my kind of humour, and I just know we are going to get on well!

The term she jokingly uses to describe herself is 'lymphomaniac'- as we breast patients need to be on our guard for our arm or hand swelling on the mastectomy side, caused by lymphodoema. This can happen at any time, even months or years later. The removal of lymph nodes interrupts the flow of lymph within the circulatory system, and fluid builds up. My nurse is passionate about it, and determined to try to help me prevent it.

It seems I had slipped through the net, and should have had such professional support from the onset. My nurse is new to this side of cancer care, but is an experienced Macmillan Nurse. She is comforting, caring and practical, and answers all my questions with truthfulness. I am so grateful to be able to place my trust in her, and she never lets me down. Although she is not involved with the chemotherapy, she often 'pops up' to the unit to support me.

I am to have six treatments, supposedly at three week intervals. The first three treatments will be one type of chemical cocktail and the last three, a different mixture of these alien cytotoxic drugs.

The first treatment of chemotherapy does not make me feel ill immediately. If it weren't for the mastectomy site, I could drive myself home. In fact, I am almost excited by it because I feel I am making strides towards recovery. It seems like a positive step. In the evening, I begin to feel a little unwell. It starts with a headache, and I can't seem to get myself up from the settee. But overall, it isn't so bad. I tell myself I can do this! It isn't so terrible after all.

As each day progresses I become more listless and tired. The tenth day onwards is less comfortable, but I feel I can cope. During the third week, I almost feel 'normal', and friends are allowed to visit. They tell me how well I look!

As another treatment passes, I expect, and get, the promised nausea and vomiting and the horrid bowel problems. Eventually my hair begins to fall out. Before this occurs, my hairdresser kindly comes to our house and cuts my hair very short, to reduce the trauma when it does happen! In reality, it isn't such a traumatic event, since I have been waiting for it. It happens in the shower after the second lot of treatment, when I am washing it. Some people find it on their pillow day after day. Mine flees en masse. It tangles like spiders' webs in my hand and ties them in knots. My husband helps me escape. As he gently smoothes the hair from my head, I slowly become bald. It is sudden.

I am to become accustomed to baldness. The wig, generously provided by the NHS, which I chose so carefully post-surgery, I do not ever wear. It is hot and itchy, and I hate it. I become adept at tying headscarves, and when the weather gets colder, I sport all kinds of hats. It's quite fun, and I can exercise my artistic side.

But as the months pass, most of the time, I go naked on top! It doesn't bother me. I am surprised to find I have a reasonably nicely shaped head, and have nothing to hide. On the very rare occasions during my months of treatment when I feel well enough to go out, my hat or scarf come off at every possible chance. My comfort is my only priority, and I am not concerned by others' reactions.   I find people are kind. Of course, many look twice, but mostly they smile, either in sympathy, or with empathy.

There are a lot of us around!

The hair loss is total for me. No eyebrows, eyelashes, and nasal hair. The latter is the uncomfortable one. My nose runs continually. But as for the rest, I don't miss the depilatory regime of old, and I'm saving a fortune on hairdresser's bills. As I have no choice, it's quite a relief, and I make the most of it!

The side effects kick in with a vengeance, with the start of the second treatment. I am so very ill, most of the time. I am told it is rare to suffer this much. I cannot eat, as I have no appetite and I feel queasy all of the time, despite the medication. Soon, I can barely get out of bed. My life revolves around existence, survival. My bedroom becomes my prison, and yet my salvation. I cannot have visitors, since my immune system is compromised. Instead, cards and flowers arrive daily, for weeks on end, and my laptop becomes my lifeline to the outside world.

A week before each treatment I have to have my blood tested at my GP's surgery, to ensure the cells have recovered sufficiently for the next dose. However, I am soon to become so ill the District Nurse attends me at home to do this. The decision was soon made by the surgery when they saw that whilst awaiting my turn, I had stretched out on a bench seat and was sound asleep. Having been called, Allan had to almost carry me into to the nurses' room. I am so weak now.

When I can eat at all, I manage very little, as my mouth always has an awful taste, and food tastes 'wrong'. Food I used to love, mainly sweet things, I can no longer tolerate. Orange juice, grapes, bananas become like poison to me. Not only do they taste awful, but also I cannot chew or swallow. As time goes on, such food that I can tolerate has to be liquidised because my mouth and throat are so ulcerated.

To make all our lives easier, certain things are, of necessity, brought in to play:

Our wonderful neighbour, a senior nurse, arranges for me to receive a Blue Badge for parking. I can no longer walk any distance at all, and it makes our lives less stressful when we attend appointments.

Essential shopping is done on line, and ironing is taken to a shop to be done. We have cleaners in once a month to do the housework and our son arranges for a friend, a local dog walker, to take care of Sandy's boundless energies – when he is not looking after me. In between all this, things often go to pot, for Allan is also trying to run his business! I can do absolutely nothing, and the family have enough to cope with.

Allan puts a notice on the front door. It politely asks visitors not to call if they have colds, coughs or worse! It may be over-protective, but it seems to work. *Of all the things that happened to me during that time, I never caught a whiff of a cold!*

Fighting cancer certainly comes at a financial cost. In our case:
> *finding different foods that I can actually eat;*
> *increased home heating costs*
> *increased costs for cooling (fans)*
> *cleaning and domestic costs*
> *hospital parking fees;*
> *travel costs (every weekday for 1 month to Tyneside)*
> *clothes appropriate for my new shape eg higher necked*
> *essential accessories such as special bras, headgear etc*
> *purchase of proprietary medicines and applications*

Allan is self employed and his earning capacity fell by 50%

There are Benefits available in certain circumstances, but alongside all the other daily survival pressures we face, the mere thought of having to go through the means-tested route is a burden we can do without. We do not pursue this avenue but know we could have called on, such as, MacMillan Cancer Support who would have advised.

≈≈≈≈≈

I am told to observe myself carefully around the tenth day post treatment, taking my temperature regularly, since this is when my white blood count will be at its lowest. I have to guard against infection, as the slightest bug can cause serious illness.

When I attended for the second treatment, I had to explain in detail the reactions I had experienced the first time round. I told the sister there had been a short period of time when my temperature had risen, and rather than call the hospital, we had taken steps to lower it – successfully.

The Unit staff did not appreciate such independent action and reminded me sternly of hidden dangers, and they once again stressed the importance of the two hour rule.

Shortly thereafter I was contacted by my Breast Nurse who lectured me, firmly but gently, about adhering to this rule and the concerns of the Unit staff that I hadn't taken their warnings seriously. I can only think this is because I am lucky enough to have a sunny nature and a smiley face. Believe me, no-one could help but take this seriously!

Oh, how all of that incident, their concerns and reprimands have been replayed in our minds since then.

We were to discover that among virtually all the professionals we had dealings with in that hospital, it was apparent that only the Chemotherapy Unit staff and the patients knew about the two hour rule.

Whenever I was subsequently admitted into hospital, no such concerns were apparent amongst the ward staff whose primary concern was always to treat me symptomatically and not take an holistic overview.

And this systemic failure was to attempt to almost kill me on two occasions.

We quickly realised that not only were we fighting cancer, we were fighting "the system"; simply, it seemed, to try to keep me alive.

THE WEB

Like a spider's web
my life looks frail;
threads tossed and blown
by the gentlest breeze,
hanging on to stems
bowing to the rain,
and elements
beyond control.

Look closer
and you will see
the hidden strength,
the interwoven tapestry
comprised of love
so gladly given
and returned,
which keeps my web
of life intact
and whole.

True enough, around the tenth day is the start of the worst time. I feel so much worse, the headaches increase, and I cannot lift my head from the pillow because of nausea. A trip to the bathroom from my bedroom is like climbing Everest. I inch my way along the landing, carefully avoiding the top of the stairs for fear of falling down them.

As time passes, my blood pressure becomes challenged, and I fall over constantly, often sliding gently to the floor to avoid damage as I feel it approaching. I am far too weak to help myself.

At the start of my five months' treatment, the weather is kind, and I can sleep in the garden during the day, Sandy lying alongside me in the shade of the awning. At other times, I have a day bed in the conservatory, when, that is, I can crawl downstairs.

When I commenced my chemotherapy, a survivor gave me some valuable advice. I repeat it throughout like a mantra, when times are so difficult for me. She said to remember that whatever happened during the treatment, it was NOT the cancer. No matter how terrible it was, I have to remember the cancer had been removed. It was such sound advice. Without it, I might have given up. If the treatment could do *this* to *me*, just imagine what it was doing to the stray cells that might have escaped during surgery.

DRIPPING

June drips away
to join the other missing months
lost in a memory of pain-filled thoughts,
supposedly a time of healing.

I aim to give myself up to it
but my aim is errant
since my trust is lost, deserting me.
How hard this is; how cruel.

Time is mapped out for me
in a rhythm beyond my choosing.
I must dance to music which jars
and jangles in my head.

Patterns forming,
life evolves outside my door,
moving, breathing, shifting,
while mine stands still and stunted.

Submission is not easy.
I want to rail and shout and scream
and make demands that can't be kept,
yet weakly I retreat and hide.

Within this lonely world
my longed-for summertime
disappears beyond my grasp
cruelly eluding me.

Resentment comes easily,
healing is invisible
trusting impossible
hoping intractable.

June will become winter
and winter brings new life;
spring, an alien memory,
summer, a forgotten barren land.

Chapter 5

THROUGH A WINDOW

The purpose of chemotherapy is to prevent cell division, thus destroying the cancer cells. Unfortunately, it cannot differentiate and prevents the production of 'good' cells too. This includes the production of blood cells, essential to life, and a careful check has to be kept on the levels of each type of blood cell. A reduction in these levels affects energy, resistance to infection, and blood clotting.

Neutropoenia is the name given to a blood condition characterised by an abnormally low number of neutrophils, a type of white blood cell. These serve to defend the body against infections by destroying bacteria in the blood. People with Neutropoenia are more susceptible to infection and, without **prompt** medical attention, the condition can be fatal.

This is known as *Neutropoenic Sepsis* and the possible deadly outcome of this condition was a key reason why the importance of the *two hour rule* had been stressed so much by the Chemotherapy Unit as well as my Breast Care Nurse.

31st July

Why is it, when you think you have been asked by 'fate' to do the hardest thing, and you do it, come through it, and survive it, you are then asked to do something far harder than you thought possible?

So hard, that the fight in you has gone; the will has gone; there is no strength left even to say, 'leave me – I'm going to live'.

I have written so much since this testing time began on April Fools' Day. Not once did I expect to say I wanted to give up. But when you have no strength left; when all you can do is curl up in a ball and drift away, you have no choice, no will of your own.

But I am lucky. The choice is left to those far stronger than I. The people who love me will not let me go. The doctor, who acknowledges immediately what is wrong with me, will not let me go. They do the fighting, and I give myself up to it as I am rushed into hospital as an emergency.

41

Seven long days later, I emerge from the hell. Seven days of others fighting and caring. I had done my fighting during the previous seven days of this truly awful episode. These seven days were theirs. They fought the battle and they won.

I am so glad to be alive, and so loved, near and far.

THE WINDOW

One square of glass;
one open window
on a different world
of leaf and twig,
of crow and earth.

And above the canopy,
the shifting clouds
and flickering light
of a sun that hides
from my view.
It tantalizes me with
shadows, sparkling
in the dew.

My mind knows it is there,
although I cannot see it.
Is that faith?
If so, then faith will
lead me to my life again,
although I cannot feel it.

(from my isolation room in hospital)

7th August

I have returned from my sojourn in hospital, and now have a little energy to reflect on the past few days.

I have had a disappointing night. I was hoping that without the perpetual call-bells ringing in my ears which I have become used to, and in view of the appalling last night spent in the Acute Medical ward, I would sleep like a log.

But I had a really awful night. I seemed to become overheated in bed, and my temperature went up, but it ended as a migraine, so all is well again. Then in the later hours, I developed a nasty cough, and couldn't get my breath, but realised that because of the throat sepsis I've not had any asthmatic inhalers for eight days. I have put that right now.

I am expecting a Macmillan Nurse today for the first time, and also a District Nurse, so I will ask them about my fluctuating temperature, since on discharge the Registrar said my white cell count, although lower than the previous night, was still high, suggesting a seat of infection somewhere. I am advised to be observant!

But once again, the system fails me.

No nurses turn up.

My head aches so much, but I don't have the strength to lift it off the pillow anyway. My temperature continues to fluctuate, and my abdomen rebels violently. I am so weak I have no strength to get to the bathroom across the landing. I lay in bed thinking, 'whom do we ring for help now, then? Who will come?'

The protocol they have is proving a complete nonsense.

And so I spend the time reflecting upon the past seven days.

I remember a friend asking at the beginning, "is your local hospital the best place for chemotherapy?" and because of all we were initially told I said yes, I was sure it was.

What we were not told was that the local hospital is only a satellite of the main Cancer Care Centre, which is in Newcastle, and therefore an Oncologist is only available in this hospital on a Wednesday!!!

You are told...."take your temperature readings seriously; people have been known to die within two hours." So to whom do you go for help when your temperature rises as they describe?

Well, the answer to that is the Chemotherapy Unit (but only on weekdays between 8.30am and 5pm). Here you have access to specialist nurses as well as one of the junior or general doctors who happens to be "on call" at the time. Thereafter, you are told to contact another specific ward.

So in my innocence at the start of it all (thinking, fool that I am...it's not going to happen to me anyway!), I assume that the designated ward is a chemotherapy specialty ward. But guess what? No, it's not; it's Haematology, which is in the right area of course, but not quite the same thing.

But I don't know that yet. At the beginning of these remarkable seven days, when my temperature rises to, and remains above, 38 degrees, we decide it is time for us to make contact. It is a Sunday afternoon. Allan phones them, and we go in expecting them to know what they are talking about, but we see a junior general doctor, one of *only four* who are covering the entire Hospital because it's the weekend. Their disinterested eyes glaze over when I name the chemicals I've been given eleven days previously. They can only look at an individual symptom and treat that.

They don't seem to be able to think holistically. So they give me potassium chloride to drink, because one of my blood test results indicates it is rather low in my body and they send me home, because, as yet, my blood levels are not critical. What they have given me to treat my low potassium chloride level, disregarding my badly ulcerated throat and mouth, is like asking me to drink the North Sea infused with razorblades. It is excruciating. I take the tablets home with me but I put them in the bin. I choose not to repeat the torture. I know it is the wrong thing to do.

Thus, I am sent home, an exercise that is repeated in the Unit during open hours, on each of the following two days, even though I can barely stagger in and Allan has to support me. I can no longer swallow. I can't drink at all. I can barely get out of bed to go there. I enter the unit by 10am and remain there in a day bed for each of the two days, until they close at 5pm. More Junior Doctors examine me and different drugs and pastes are issued to treat my throat.

Although I now have nine adverse symptoms, they attempt to treat only the worst – my ulcerated mouth and throat. My temperature fluctuates from one extreme to the other but no one looks at "me" – just my mouth and throat. On my third day of this ordeal, a knowledgeable Macmillan Nurse visits me in the Unit. Again, she focuses on my worst symptom and immediately consigns to the bin the still unopened drugs so recently issued by the Junior Doctor! She is able to prescribe something that eventually makes a difference, but by then my downward spiral has been ordained.

At the end of day three and as Allan prepares to take me home (using his mother's wheelchair to get me to the car), the Ward Sister tells him I "should really be admitted to a ward" and then adds..."but there isn't a bed to be had in the entire hospital".

This, we feel, seems to be a perpetual state within this supposed flagship of the Private Finance Initiative/Health Service system, where the hospital (and many like it) is underfunded, under-staffed and does not have the capacity to cope with demand. Opened in April 2001 with much fanfare, it was only weeks later that reports of "not fit for purpose" illustrations were being released to the media by senior consultants, administrators and nurses. Not least among the problems was that of bed capacity. Among many journalists of the time, the Guardian feature writer, Felicity Lawrence, closely followed events and in a lengthy article about our new hospital, wrote "like other similar PFIs around the country... has fewer beds than the hospitals it replaces. The scheme emerged after many revisions from an original plan going back to 1991 to centralise services for the area in a new district general hospital with 798 beds. This plan involved downgrading a neighbouring hospital...in the County. But when the final business case for the new building was drawn up, the plans were for 454 beds". From almost 1,000 available beds between the two hospitals, there eventually emerged a total of only 591. Is it any wonder that the Hospital is always operating at full bed capacity?

I spend the fourth day in my own bed, my family constantly monitoring me vigilantly, but on day five my condition worsens appreciably and I now have to be pushed into the hospital in a wheelchair. I lie curled up on a ward bed waiting, (wanting), to die, drifting in and out of consciousness. But on this occasion I am triaged as I am wheeled onto the ward and am obviously regarded as being in a critical condition so am lucky enough to be seen immediately and treated by a wonderful (junior) doctor who takes an holistic view, and just by luck, my life is saved. She told Allan that a further thirty minutes delay would have been fatal. By then, I was past caring.

And the luck holds, because I am put (in my opinion) in the best ward of the hospital...not only because they have the only isolation room available in the entire hospital, but also because basic nursing standards and discipline are so evident. That Junior Doctor (and Allan) saved my life. She was just at the end of her first year, and left two days later to do required GP training rotation.

The entire batch of Junior Doctors left on the same day, to be replaced by new ones, straight out of medical school, with no experience at all, other than their training and their brand new qualification.

Little did I then know that this factor would feature in my life shortly after.

But my seven days as an in-patient puts me back on the right track again! I am well cared for in my isolated room. My veins, in protest, finally accept the canular and urgently needed antibiotics of several kinds are administered the whole time; observations are taken, and my difficult diet is catered for. Since I cannot eat the routine meals provided because of my food allergies, the restaurant chef provides my food, and a member of staff collects each meal for me. In fact, I can eat very little, because my mouth is so ulcerated. I am as awkward as Allan explained to the Oncologist I would be, and we have no doubt that 'my awkwardness' is behind my adverse reactions to the chemotherapy.

The seven days feel like a month, and I am delighted when I am told I can finally go home. For some strange reason, two Registrars from different departments visit me within the space of an hour. One tells me I must follow protocol for my condition and wait the usual twenty-four hours post antibiotics before being allowed home. The next one tells me I can leave immediately. Stupidly, I don't question this anomaly. Instead, I delight in the fact that I can at last leave. Hindsight suggests, of course, that my room was needed for another patient, hence my speedy discharge.

So guess what happens next? Only three hours after being discharged from hospital and coming home, my temperature rises again, I begin to feel ill, and in trepidation, we follow the dictated protocol again.

Allan makes many phone calls, but there are no beds available on the haematology ward and sadly not on my recently vacated ward either. So they say I have to go in to A&E, and on our arrival Allan is advised to immediately direct me to the Acute Medical ward where they are now expecting me.

It is our personal experience, confirmed by many people to whom we have spoken, that this ward just happens to be the busiest one in the hospital. As an Acute Medical Admissions ward, patients usually stay for a night or two for assessment, and to be stabilised, and then are moved to the most appropriate ward for their condition. It is always full to the brim with some thirty or so very sick people, with all kinds of conditions, and presumably, all kinds of bugs.

I cannot get out of the car; I am no longer capable of even holding myself up. I'm wheeled in to the Hospital, into A&E and then along to the ward, by paramedics. At the Nurses' Station, a bed number is given, and I am taken to a four bedded open room where there are three other patients.

Now *we* can see the nonsense of this... I've just come from total isolation... so I refuse to allow them to push me into the area. They are confounded that someone can be so stroppy!! I'm wheeled back to the Nurses' Station, where we are assured that the patients in the four bedded ward are non-infectious (oh really?? –one just had to listen to the chesty coughs of two of the occupants to question that assurance). But I reluctantly agree to stay, since (surprise, surprise) apparently it's the only bed available in the entire hospital.

It is now 10pm; I have a temperature, and am utterly exhausted.

As I am put into the bed, we notice that a lady in the adjoining, curtained-off bed is calling for assistance. Her calls go unheard, or unheeded, by the nurse who, at 10 30pm, does my observations. And yes, protocol demands that I be treated as a new admission. Allan suggests my medical notes be obtained from the ward I had left, a little over 4 hours earlier but the nurse tells him no one is available to collect them from that ward. He offers to do so but is told that "patient confidentiality" will not allow him to handle them. She has to leave me for a few minutes and Allan decides to visit my previous ward and seek their help in providing the records. He found they already knew about me being re-admitted and the Sister immediately instructed a nurse to find the file and accompany him back to the new ward and hand them over to my new Staff Nurse.

We can understand the complexity of issues relating to "confidentiality" but can't help but think that in situations such as this, "the system" supersedes the well-being of the patient.

My 'urgent' observations and bloods are finally completed by the Staff Nurse at 11pm, and my temperature continues to rise (as does my temper!). Now I wait to be assessed by a Junior Doctor whose first day *ever* this is on a Ward as a qualified doctor! But there are other admissions to be seen before me.

My neighbour continues to call for assistance. She uses the call button but it goes unanswered. Allan walks along the corridor to find a nurse, without success. There are only three on duty and one is on her break, leaving only two – and this is a busy Medical Admissions ward.

By 1 40am, *(you remember the dire two hour warning?)* having rung our daughter to bring my digital thermometer in, and Allan then recording my half hourly observations, I think..........'I know I am in the worst possible place. My temperature is now decreasing, but still fluctuates madly from one extreme to the other. I would be safer at home'. So we pack up my things, and Allan assists me to the exit, just as a nurse appears in the corridor. To her utter disbelief, I announce "I am going home". Boy, does that put the cat among the pigeons! She cannot believe it as I walk out into the corridor! She asks Allan to remain for a few minutes and he explains precisely why we consider it unsafe for me to remain. He is assured I will be seen quickly and I am eventually persuaded that I "will be seen by a Doctor within ten minutes".

He finds me in the corridor, and I reluctantly return to the ward where the calls of my neighbour are weaker now and, soon after, we start to hear and then see the trickle of urine as she finally gives up hope of ever being helped.   Allan manages to find a nurse and she comes to see the lady who, it transpires has been sitting in a chair for the past several hours. It is now the early hours of the morning. She is blind and cannot walk unaided, and she is distressed that such a thing could happen to her. The nurse talks to her in condescending tone – and we want to shout and rail against the indignity inflicted upon that poor lady by the systemic failures of this under-staffed and under-resourced hospital.

It is now 2am (almost 5 hours after my re-admission) and I am back in my bed, and the on call Junior Doctor, on his *very* first day finally comes to assess me. We kindly make it easier for him, and dictate most of the details, anticipate his questions, and remind him of those he's missed! He is very grateful. The reason I've had to wait so long is because (you remember?) it's his first day, they are very busy and he is rather slow!

So much for the two-hour rule- *which he has never heard of* – until now!

Then, finally, the Registrar arrives. It is almost 3am *(remember the two hour warning? -* It is now six hours later!)   However, thankfully, she is sound and sensible. We accept her assurance that none of the staff are to blame for this debacle. She tells us it is" the organisation" – leaving us to add "in this 'wonderful' new understaffed and under-funded supposed Flagship hospital". And to think that the, then, Prime Minister extolled the virtues of the Private Funding Initiative scheme   Oh, that he would agree to be a "patient-in-disguise" here for just 48hours. Am I getting too political?

I agree to stay in until the morning, since my blood is not normal. Contrarily, I now have a high white cell count, and it needs to be tested again. Luckily, although it is still a problem in the morning (whilst I am no longer Neutropoenic, it shows I may have an infection...but no-one knows where) I am allowed home.........since, I am told, it is the safest place for me!! Before I leave, I cut up the blind lady's breakfast, and help her to eat. No-one else is around to do it.

But what next?? My first night home, and in my own bed, I start getting hot again, and I lie there thinking 'where do I go? Whom do I call?' Luckily, I think, it is only a migraine.

But I have two more treatments to go, albeit my Oncologist decides these should be of a reduced dose, and with a special injection to try to prevent the dramatic downturn in my condition. But I now have the constant and very daunting thought: - how can I possibly trust my life to this hospital?

If there is any good to come from these past two dreadful weeks, it is that we were invited to a meeting of involved staff, to air our concerns, and to commit them in writing.

Having done that, we later heard that our experiences were then used as a case study during a Chemotherapy Unit staff training session. Hopefully others will not be subjected to the same sufferings, but we have our doubts. The training is really needed on the wards where patients such as me, who are adversely affected by chemotherapy, are admitted, and where no Oncologist is available to provide specialist input.

*My plea to them remains unchanged. It is this: **listen to the patient.** We may not fit all your criteria, and tick all your boxes, but we really do know our bodies best. If we tell you there is something wrong, please, please believe us!*

At home, a few days later, in my weakened state, I suffer a slipped disc, doing something as simple as trying to get out of a chair. I am in agony, and one of our GPs comes to my rescue. I cannot sit or stand. I can just lie on the floor, or crawl to the sofa, which now becomes my bed. That poor GP! It is just his luck to be on-call for home visits! By this stage, we are all "struggling". Mum- in- law, now living with us, is becoming increasingly frail and requires constant care. Despite visits from Carers four times each day, there is still much that Allan has to do for her. I can do nothing for myself, and our daughter has also become quite poorly. This is one of our lowest times- and the GP sits with us for an hour, listening to our tales and rails, and quietly responding. We are his final call of the day and although, as he tells us, his evening meal is ready for him at home, he knows he will not return to work for forty-eight hours. On leaving us, he returns to the surgery and writes a detailed brief for all his colleagues. Over the next few days, they regularly telephone to enquire how things are.

Fortunately for me, the painful back spasms pass in a few days, and I get better relatively quickly. Something else for which to be grateful! My General Practice has been so supportive. We only have to make a phone-call, and they respond to our requests.

I am beginning to feel more comfortable in my mastectomy site, and I decide the time is right to be fitted with my prosthesis. The word amuses me, and conjures up the image in my mind of a false leg. Infantile humour, which pleases me! I picture it, the painted false toes peeping out of the top of my blouse as I reach the top notes in an imaginary concert in the distant future. I am not safe to be let loose with the word 'prosthesis'! To me this is, and always will be, a false booby!

My Breast Care Nurse calls at my house, her bag of false boobies with her! They come in their own cushioned boxes sitting in padded cradles to prevent them from wrinkling and misshaping. I am told it has to be kept in the box when not in use. I find that part a little odd to deal with. In the privacy of my bedroom, and with much humour, it is an easy transition to become double-breasted again. We have already discussed the size I used to be, and we now spend much care in matching it with the remaining one. I don't want to over-balance! My wonderful nurse makes it a fun procedure. For many women this can be a tricky time. As always, my nurse matches her humour to mine, as we parade in front of the mirror, checking the equality of size, her experienced hand and eye assessing me. I have to don a t-shirt which she tightens at the back to test for size and appearance. I feel like a page 3 model! Tears are in my eyes, but not for the loss, but from the laughter. Today is all about hugs and laughter and tears, and the future is not discussed.

As a reward, I stick an extra gold heart on my survivor's chart.

THE STORM

The storm is nearly over.
The fiercest battle
may yet be won.
The garden is deserted;
flowers lie
scattered at her feet.

Petals, battered by tears,
fall silently
to wither in the sun
from where they cannot rise
but fade away.
Sadness is complete.

The lark no longer rises
as when she was
unknowing and young.
Buds drop from their stems,
leaves fall,
paths no longer meet.

But the storm is nearly over.
New songs
await her to be sung.
The garden just lies dormant;
resting, waiting,
familiar, precious and sweet.

Neutropoenic Sepsis

When my neutropoenic sepsis diagnosis was given to us, Allan immediately researched the condition online, for neither of us really knew much about it. As part of that research, he came across a book entitled "Breast Cancer", written by a Consultant Surgeon. We have not sought his permission to include the following extract but trust he will accept our grateful thanks for providing this incredibly valuable guide which, for people in our situation at that time, proved essential:

"Breast Cancer"
By

J Michael Dixon, MD
Edinburgh Breast Unit, Western General Hospital

"Neutropoenic infection, or sepsis, is responsible for a significant proportion of life threatening events and should be anticipated and, when suspected, treated aggressively and promptly"

As you can imagine, those words rang alarm bells in Allan's mind and he immediately copied, pasted and printed the above extract onto a small card which he then carried in his wallet at all times.

Since the author of this, and several other related books, is a Consultant Surgeon at the Edinburgh Breast Unit, one might assume his opinion would be respected within the medical community.

Not so within our local hospital.

When need arose, only one of several doctors and nurses who were shown the quote by way of flagging up the potential threat of Neutropoenia, actually took it seriously. Each of the others responded in differing ways. Some clearly thought Allan was questioning their professional skills; others took it from him, but did not read it; two nurses patronisingly told him not to worry, the doctors (when they finally arrived) would know what they were doing. One doctor read it and laughed. We were not privy to the reason for his amusement.

Of course, apart from the one who took note of what was written, the others contributed to wasting valuable time in diagnosing my condition and to increasing my suffering, whilst Allan fought to protect my life.

We make the suggestion to Health Service policy makers that a small, business sized, card bearing the (above) extract from Michael Dixon's book should be inserted into every chemotherapy patient's "red book". If it then becomes necessary for a patient to be admitted to A&E or to a Ward, on admission they, or their carer, can produce that card and immediately alert staff to consider the presence or onset of Neutropoenic Sepsis and serve as a reminder that early and aggressive intervention is required.

11th September   ^{4am}

The end of this stage of my long adventure does not come quickly. Even on this last day of chemotherapy, my sleep the night before is broken and short.

My head replays scenes from the stage of the Chemotherapy Unit theatre; scenes I would rather forget. But I cannot forget, and nor can I sleep. I am haunted by fears that today will not be my last day here....that one day I will have to return. I repeat all the positive things I have been told about my own condition, and I know I am being foolish. But my brain is beyond my control at four o'clock in the morning.

But today is a positive day. What could be better than entering that door for the last time? The last soaking of my hand in a bowl of hot water to encourage shattered veins to offer themselves one last time; the last canular to be inserted to deliver necessary poison into my already poisoned body?

Months ago, on my first day, as I sat waiting, I wrote the 'Courage' poem. How right I was! I have needed every ounce of courage within me, and from others who have supported, loved and inspired me along the way.

And how I needed that love, inspiration and support! It will not surprise those who know me well, that my physical rebellion against those cytotoxic drugs would be one of the 'worst cases known" to the Unit staff. Was that, I wonder, to make them/me feel better? Was it a stock phrase in the "how to deal with difficult patients" staff manual? Surely there must be others like me? Indeed, we went on to meet some and hear their stories. Some did not survive.

Anyway, why would I take the valley when I can climb over impassable mountains?

One more treatment to face and it will soon be over.

SAFETY

Morning comes;
mellow secrets slip silently away
to leave behind the whisper of a song,
the brush of a soft wing.

And at the water's edge
inside her mind
he, who thought she did the leading,
leads her to the safety of a harbour.

Like the mermaid trapped by weeds
she lies ensnared forever in his mind,
no showy butterfly of colour and light,
but the strength of the bees' wing.

As I wait for the time to pass to leave for my very last chemotherapy treatment, I cannot believe this long awaited day is here. Bring it on!! I am ready for you. And as you try to sicken me, hurt me, and beat me down during the next three weeks, I will cross off each day knowing I have beaten *you*, and won.

I have never been competitive or combatant. I have never needed to come first. It does give me pride and satisfaction that the things I love doing, I do well – working with children, painting (well, sometimes!!), singing, and writing my poetry.

But this is a battle I have been determined to win, and nothing less will do. I will never give in to it – not the disease, or the painful methods used to destroy that disease.

This is *my* time and fate will not be allowed to take it away from me. It may seem it has taken a year from my life, but it hasn't. It has changed and altered the year for all of us, not just for me, but also for all those who love me. But it has *not* taken it.

From it, I have learned about myself and about others around me. It has made me aware of the great privilege of knowing how much I am loved.

From it, I have found my weaknesses and strengthened them; found my strengths and shared them.

So no fate, you did not steal my year. Nor shall you steal the rest of my life.

And here I sit, back in the same waiting area, waiting and waiting. Why give so many appointments for the same times? The nurses dash from one patient to another, ceaselessly. Phones ring; people chatter; pumps attached to drips sound alarms. Dispiritingly, some of these pumps have little plaques on them. I assume they are 'in memoriam' dedications to past patients, but maybe they are also from grateful patients. I am grateful not to have to use one of these.

There is no privacy and no peace.

People tell me their stories..........some I really don't want to hear.

When I can, I close my eyes and disappear into myself while I wait. Does determination give you choice? I am determined to live, to fulfil my promised future. I want this to be an end to the evil that silently invaded my body.

Let *this* be an end to it.

Chapter 6

COCOONED

29th September

And so the second chapter of this unexpected, unwanted story draws to a close, as dramatically as it started. And here I am in hospital again. Another Neutropoenia and another emergency admission.

My final treatment has had the last laugh.

I fought to stay at home, but admission became inevitable. Yet this time we know the system! We know what treatment to demand, and, in theory, we now know how to get it quickly. I say 'we', but in fact, I am once again past helping myself. I can no longer fight; I lie on my bed at home waiting to die, but Allan will not let me. I have slept badly and by 5am I already know what is happening within my body.

As I write this now, Allan has to remind me what happened next, since I was beyond conscious thought.

I woke Allan and he then followed due process and at intervals took my temperature and monitored my condition. An hour later, he contacted the emergency GP service which is actually located within the hospital.

Having outlined my condition, the duty nurse advised she would find my file and the Doctor would call back within twenty minutes. For Allan that became a very long and terrible twenty minutes.

The return call was made; further discussions took place and just minutes later, a wonderful GP had arrived and was examining me in my bed. She understood my needs at once and the associated urgency.

She took blood samples and her driver immediately delivered them to the pathology laboratory. She also spent much time trying to find me an isolation room but, of course, none were available, and so we were told to get to the hospital quickly where a bed was being prepared on the designated ward for chemotherapy related patients.

Allan wheels me onto that ward but they immediately usher us through more doors and we find ourselves entering the adjoining ward– where I had spent my first Neutropoenic isolation.

By way of greeting, I am brusquely and unkindly told by the admitting nurse that another very ill patient has been ejected from this room to make way for me – she gives us both the impression that she feels too much fuss is being made on my behalf! But I can feel no guilt, for once again I am struggling to live. Neither of us responds to this unprofessional comment. We have both been thrust back into the battle for my survival and now is not the time to take issue. Neither of us has the energy to spare.

It might be assumed that notice would have been taken of the emergency GP's report and the accompanying pathology blood test results produced 2/3 hours earlier in this hospital's own laboratory, but – no! That procedure is not in the handbook - apparently.

I am put into bed – and left. It is now four hours since the GP visited, she having remained with me for almost three hours. She knew the two hour rule and was staying close by until I could be hospitalised. She was a gem!

Despite a GP report and the path lab result, no account of either is taken when I am assessed. We are then left alone in the room. Having learnt by previous experience, Allan has brought in with him my digital thermometer, pen and paper and he records thirty minute readings as per prescribed protocol. The record shows that, as usual, my temperature fluctuates from one extreme to the other.

Almost three hours after admission, my temperature rapidly rises and remains elevated. I continue to be assailed by rigors* and I descend once again into that distant place where I seek only peace. No one has been back to the room to check on me throughout that period of time. Allan cannot find a member staff anywhere, and eventually kicks up a fuss by calling for help in the corridor outside my room. Someone appears and he is condescendingly told by a Staff Nurse that there is another patient along the corridor with a much higher temperature than mine! Allan, a man of infinite patience, loses it, pointing out that the diagnoses are most likely very different. I can do nothing but curl up in a ball and submit to my fate. I can no longer even speak for myself.

*('a rigor is an episode of shaking or exaggerated shivering which can occur with a high fever. It is an extreme reflex response, which occurs for

a variety of reasons. It should not be ignored as it is often a marker for significant and sometimes serious infections'.....Patient UK)

Things suddenly start to happen; a doctor finally comes to see me, and I am quickly surrounded by nurses, each doing essential observations to record my rapidly deteriorating condition. The prescribed regime is followed to the letter – albeit reactively and against the ticking clock.

Allan becomes more concerned by my quickening deterioration and the insistence of the staff that due process must be carried out to the letter from the beginning, including a full social history (such as: how many bathrooms do we have in our house; do we have central heating?) As if they hadn't gathered the same information about me so many times previously! As I cannot provide any coherent responses, a nurse takes Allan to one side to complete the paperwork and, he thinks, to remove him from the frantic activity now taking place around me.

Moments later he notices my condition is now deteriorating very rapidly, he intervenes and tells the doctor she must telephone my Oncologist for instructions.

Clearly, this causes consternation, for within the "NHS system", there are strict hierarchical protocols – and here was a patient's relative demanding that things be done *his* way and definitely contravening both protocol and policy.

He wins the day for, after my previous Neutropoenic episode, my Consultant Oncologist had given us some direct telephone numbers which could be used to contact either her or her Registrar if ever there was the need. Confident in that knowledge, Allan stands directly in front of the Junior Doctor and taps out one of the numbers on his mobile phone, at which point the doctor quickly reaches the decision that she should phone the Oncologist herself.

Immediately following that call, a canular is inserted, with the usual extreme difficulty, (even unsuccessfully attempting to insert them into my feet on previous occasions) and the intravenous antibiotics are finally started. My veins and the surrounding tissue are very compromised due to the chemotherapy, and of course, my mastectomy arm must not be used. It takes a very skilled person to even get a canular in now. However, it is now eight hours since the emergency duty GP took a blood sample, and diagnosed a severe Neutropoenic level of 0.01%.

"The system" apparently does not allow for acceptance of the GP's diagnosis, even though it had been substantiated by a pathology report produced within this same hospital just five hours earlier. If that laboratory report had been accepted, my treatment could have started five hours earlier than it eventually did. In the event, from first seeing the on-call Doctor to commencing treatment, nine hours had elapsed. Is this an area for a protocol review?

Remember the two hour warning and the concern by members of the Chemotherapy Unit that they considered *I* might not take it seriously?

Once again, Allan's care, determination and promptness save me and I am cocooned again, in my isolation room.

COCOONED

Autumn slips in quietly
behind cold glass,
to the sound of
cawing quarrels overhead,
and the hum
of others' normal lives.

No wind on my face,
shielded in my cocoon
behind blind faith.
Nothing touches me,
just my own drama
acted out on a stage of isolation.

And through a door
forbidden to me,
others act out their own plays.
Curtains fall, never to rise again,
while others fight for freedom.

I prefer glass for now.

(from my isolation room window I have a view of a rookery, which becomes my lifeline)

59

After the now-to-be-expected debacle of my admission, I am well cared for once again. My condition rapidly improves after the first twenty-four hours of intravenous antibiotics. I spend my isolation time in a well-remembered pattern. A lot of my time is spent curled up in a chair by the open window observing the antics of the squirrels and rooks. My days pass in now typical routine. Drips are constantly changed, sometimes well into the night hours; observations are taken with competent regularity; drugs are issued; blood tests taken, and little meals brought in by Allan often provide my midnight feast. My night nurses are particularly caring, and cheer with me when finally my blood test is returned recording that I am past the danger level. I put a large sign up on the wall noting my score in Olympic skating fashion, and each nurse who comes in rejoices with me. As always in hospital, each day seems like three, and another week passes in this fashion. It is soporific and strangely restful.

This time the Hospital's Bed Management does not intervene and I am not discharged until all traces of infection have disappeared and not until (as in good old fashioned nursing days) my antibiotic drips had been removed for at least twenty-four hours (unlike my first neutropoenic episode).

I am home, and very weak. Unable to walk or care for myself in any way at all, friends step in to look after me during the times Allan stays at the hospital with his mother, who had been admitted as I was discharged. I am not sure how my poor husband is surviving this terrible time himself!

Over a period of the past few years, our many experiences, both personal and familial, of the understaffed and under-resourced Acute Medical Admissions Ward display some of the worst of services that our local hospital can provide, despite the best efforts of the dedicated, but weary, overstretched staff. We were to discover it could be even worse than our previous experiences.

As a flagship PFI/NHS facility, it really is quite appalling across so many areas of patient care – and as this is being written, the news has focussed on three hospitals in different parts of the country, which have been found similarly wanting, if not worse. We can certainly empathise with patients in those hospitals.

Having the mastectomy was the easy part, I have found. I coped with that well I think, but only with the help and boosting self confidence of those who love me. This second part has been truly awful. In my hospital room I have just been told by my Oncologist *'Chemotherapy doesn't agree with you.'* Understatement!!!

Almost six months, and six treatments later, and I am told chemotherapy doesn't really agree with me, although of course I realise it has been an evil necessity!! Out of those six months, only three separate weeks have been bearable. The rest have been spent in my bed, on a makeshift bed in the conservatory, or in a hospital bed.

Every week, every hour, every moment, has been spent in various shades of hell, known only to those closest to me, without whom I would not have survived to reach this stage. At first, I thought I must be weak, or spineless, since so many others who have been through chemotherapy have said they managed to 'pull round' after a few days and get on with life, albeit restricted. It was a relief in the end to find I was in fact 'different.'

As with my breast, the vanity side has not troubled me enormously. You quickly come to terms with being completely hairless, and single breasted, when those you love are totally unaffected, and you know you are loved for simply being you.

But the isolating pain and torment of an adverse reaction to chemotherapy - as opposed to normal side effects - has been a nightmare I would never wish to repeat. I thought I would not get through it. Many times, I wailed 'I can't do this again.' However, I wasn't allowed to get away with that, luckily! My nurse/friend/neighbour, as she puffed up my pillows and made me comfortable at home in Allan's absence when he was caring for his Mum, would remind me of the times I had said it before, but had always gone on to do it again....and again. Quite true, but how glad I am it's over.

Meanwhile

Our lives have rarely been straightforward, and nothing changes now. Such was the constancy of the battle I have been fighting, we all now felt trapped in a never ending cycle of dramatic circumstances.

As if the onset of my second Neutropoenic episode were not enough, there was more with which to contend.

In the short time that it took the Out of Hours (hospital based) Emergency Doctor to respond by telephone to Allan's initial appeal for help for me during my second Neutropoenic episode, his ninety year- old mother, who had moved in with us a few weeks earlier, tried to get out of bed on her own and had fallen. When the doctor arrived, she found she had two patients, both named Susan Percival!

The elder Mrs P disappeared off in the ambulance with our daughter accompanying her, whilst I was taken by car to be admitted to hospital! At that stage, she had not seen me at all so, as Allan wheeled me into the hospital in Mum's wheelchair, we diverted via the A&E Dept to allow a moment for her to see I was actually alive and to grasp my hand for a moment.

Mum was not admitted to a ward at that time, and she returned home a few hours later, having sustained serious bruising to her shoulder. Allan and our family then had to combine visiting me in hospital whilst providing additional care and support for Mum.

Three weeks later

The fall added to her increasing frailty and she had to be admitted three weeks later into the infamous (for our family, and subsequently we have seen and heard of many similar tales of woe) Acute Medical ward where it was discovered she had recently suffered a slight heart attack. This was all part of her continuing decline in physical health.

In this ward, she was treated with such indignity and appalling neglect, that Allan had to remain by her bedside for many hours just to ensure her care and safety. This was my eighth day, post chemo, and once again, I was very poorly and confined to bed. I was left in the capable hands of friends and neighbours whilst Allan sat with his mother in the hospital ward.

As he wheeled her onto the ward, a water jug was hurled from a unit, into the corridor, just ahead of them. Minutes later, they discovered that the only bed available on the ward was in this same mixed four bedded unit that included a highly disorientated, foul mouthed and violent man who required constant monitoring and restraint. His repeated attempts to exit the ward showed that this monitoring was not completely successful. Not only did Mum find it acutely embarrassing to be in a mixed bay (two male and two females) she was also intimidated by the man who was in the opposite bed. Worse still, three hours later, there were then three men in the bay and eventually she was moved to an adjacent, ladies only, bay.

Since arriving in that bay, it had then taken three (ignored) requests by Allan for a large volume of splattered blood and other fluids of the previous bed-occupant to be washed away from Mum's bedside cabinet and surrounding floor area. It was only when, almost two hours later, he went to the Sister and asked for access to gloves and cleaning materials so that he could remove the detritus, that a nurse was directed to clean the mess.

Five hours after being admitted, Mum was seen by a very new junior doctor. He was obviously "rushed off his feet" and immediately started talking to Mum whilst, at the same time looking down at her file to read her notes. Allan tried to interrupt him but the medic was clearly "on a roll", at the end of which he expected to receive an answer from Mum. Instead, she turned to Allan and asked "What did he say?" The Doctor then appeared to listen to Allan's explanation that he should look at her as he was speaking and direct his voice towards the hearing aid microphone which lay on her chest. He told Allan not to worry as he'd been trained to communicate with deaf people and knew what to do, upon which he then leant over, so that his mouth was very close to Mum's left ear, and bellowed "HELLO, I'M DOCTOR XXX, CAN YOU TELL ME WHERE YOU HAVE THE PAIN?"

Mum did not flinch, for she had no hearing in her left ear at all (by courtesy of a German bomb in 1944). She was feeling dreadful and she shrugged her shoulders in exasperation. Allan just laughed in despair at the doctor's stupidity – but there was no time for further discussion as a bleep sounded and Doctor XXX was promptly called away before any examination could be started.

He returned more than an hour later but, as before, he was called away to a more urgent case, having only had time to once again bellow in her ear "HELLO, I'M DOCTOR XXX". His third visit was even briefer, for no sooner had he pulled the curtain around Mum's bed than a patient in a bed opposite had a heart attack, and he was called away by her relatives. Mum had been admitted to the ward at lunchtime and it wasn't until 9.30pm that she was finally seen by a doctor – this time, a Registrar.

Allan returned home at 10.30pm, having had a constant round of medical situations to contend with since 5.00am, and filled with concern both for having left me for so long and also for leaving his vulnerable mother behind in that ward to fend for herself. The following morning he returned to the hospital at 9.30am, to discover Mum in a very distressed state. She had a very frail body and she could not walk or manoeuvre herself, but her mind was very alert and she was fully aware of all that was happening around her. Being unable to attract the attention of a nurse, she was now lying in faeces.

A new drip had been inserted at 7am (according to her chart) but it had not been connected securely and the much needed anti-biotic fluid was discharging into her bed, so she was also lying in wet bedding. When the drip was applied, she told the nurse she urgently required the toilet and was informed someone would return to assist her. No one had been near her since then and her calls went unanswered. Those who did the breakfast round heard her decline any food because she really needed to use the toilet. They had said they would return after the breakfast round, but they never did and her pleas for help were ignored.

Having organised that she be immediately attended to, Allan's remonstrations to the Ward Sister led to him being introduced to the Sister-Manager of the ward who agreed there had been failings in the standard of care provided for his mother. He was told that the past twenty-four hours had been a "once in a year" occurrence when everything conspired to test the resources of the ward.

Allan pointed out that we had already experienced three or four such "one-off" occurrences in this very ward within the past few months!

In common with so many of her colleagues, she conveyed exasperation that "the system" prevented the staff from providing good patient care and urged that he write to the Health Trust because, hopefully, more notice would be taken of comments by patients/carers than by frontline staff.

WILD FLOWERS

The memories come in batches now,
reminding me of how things were
and how they might have been.
How the mind plays tricks.

The garden withers and flowers fade
and weeds spring up and thrive instead,
ensnaring shallow roots.
How the heart deceives.

But what are weeds, but flowers wild,
less fragile than the ones before,
with beauty of their own?
How a garden thrives.

And we will plant and we will grow,
as we have done in days gone by,
with beauty of our own.
How a garden heals.

Chapter 7

JOINING THE DOTS

30th September

The next chapter is about to open for me, radiotherapy. Let us hope I am not a unique specimen in that area too!

I do NOT wish to go down in Medical History books.

I just want to be normal.

What is it about a diagnosis of cancer that causes commonsense and intelligence to fly out of the window?

I find myself asking inane questions of the professionals, when I already know the sensible answers. Yet my head devises scenarios beyond my control.

It is the fear of having everything you know, everything you *are*, snatched away from you, when all you want is your old life back. You don't want more; you just want to be you again.

And so the third phase begins. A trip to Newcastle involves the discovery that I am unable to walk properly yet! The autumn sun is on my face. It too, is weaker now, but I still return with more freckles along with the tattoos, (sorry to disappoint again.....no butterfly on my bum.....although I did ask for one!). The tattoos are essential to identify the areas for radiation. I am told some people fret about these minute permanent marks, and that they can eventually be removed by laser, but they shall be my little badges of courage! It amuses me to think I might concern myself with these minute dots, when I have an eight inch scar across my chest, and a few hundred more freckles on my face now.

I have been allowed out of the isolation room in one hospital to keep this initial appointment in another, but I am taken by wheelchair to a small room, as far away from other people as possible. The vast open waiting room is filled with patients and their companions. Wigs and scarves abound!

66

The scan is made easy for me, with two radiographers explaining everything. It is not diagnostic (as we all fear) but a preparation for the next phase. The tattooing is not painful. It is just typical, and unfortunate for me, that the oral antibiotics I started this morning begin to rebel! I am vomiting.

Should I ever expect otherwise? I have one week before treatment begins. Will I be lucky enough to make it a fourth good week in six months?

≈≈≈≈≈

Well how silly of me to think it may be easy!!

I do have a week off in between the change of chemotherapy and radiotherapy treatments, but in that interval, I develop a frozen shoulder which is so painful it is almost unendurable. Luckily (?) it is in the opposite shoulder to my mastectomy side. Ironically, I have conducted my physiotherapy on my mastectomy side assiduously, and it is flexible and fluid. I wake myself up every night, whimpering with the pain in my sleep. I have to attend for physiotherapy sessions, and eventually have an injection into the shoulder at my local doctor's surgery. This is painful, but thankfully does the trick.

TIME ON MY HANDS

It yawns chasm-like ahead of me;
gapes behind me.
Helplessly I bow to its dictates,
weakly acknowledging its hold over me.
It gives me no choice.

And yet, what is it?
Is it the passing of an hour, a day-
yet another moment in the blinking of my life?

It is all my emotions
crumpled together,
tossed and cushioned in a soft blanket of warmth,
tender and secret,
silently acknowledged only to myself
and sometimes to another;
quietly enduring,
stretching and yawning like a new-born thought.

Time is irrelevant,
just the ticking of a clock
I cannot, will not, ever hear.

14th October

This is my first visit to the new Northern Centre for Cancer Care in Newcastle. It only opened the day before, and I expect teething problems, but from the moment we park the car and walk through the revolving doors of this magnificent multi-million pound building, I feel safe.

As I am greeted and meet the staff, I feel I am secure for the first time since I left the private hospital, post mastectomy. Amazingly the staff are so competent, and I feel at once that I can hand myself over to them. This is a vast difference from the feeling I have had in the past six months; the need to check everyone and everything that is done to me rapidly disappears. It is a huge relief.

My room is called Room 7. At present, it feels a bit like Orwell's Room 101 to me, as the fear of the future never leaves me. Yet I know I am in a Centre of Excellence. The room, of course, is grandly brand new, like the rest of the building, which is almost empty of patients. It is such an impressive building; airy, spacious and well designed. Our footsteps echo in the empty corridors, and smart new chairs sit empty; water fountains stand idle waiting for the first drops to fall; toilets are unused, pristine; wards await future patients, and the cafe we pass on the way in has an air of expectancy about it. The Centre will not be fully operational for another few months so I am privileged to be among the first to attend here, while it is sparkling new.

I am ushered into a changing room and given a dark blue 'uniform' to put on, a complex arrangement of Velcro and zip which is very difficult to don (especially with a frozen shoulder!), but makes manoeuvring me easy for the crew, once on the table! It is mine for the duration, to take home, and carry back and forth every day. It is stiff, and it smells and feels brand new.

I am to have twenty sessions of treatment, five days a week for a month, but the first day is to go over the measurements taken the previous week at the old department. Sadly for me, all the measurements now need adjusting, probably because of my shoulder, and because of the intense pain, the radiographer suggests waiting a further week. But I feel unable to wait, I am geared up for this, and I want to get it over. After the delays with Neutropoenia, I don't want to risk waiting another week. I assure them I can bear the pain, and they go ahead. Fine brave words! As I lie on the table, and am manoeuvred into position, the tears run into my bald scalp and I grit my teeth.

If it weren't my body on the table, the fascination of the technology would enthral me. Everything is large, agile and mobile - the table, and the machine looming above me. I receive further tiny tattoos, and am liberally marked with felt tip pens, the marks becoming my badge of office over the coming weeks. I look like a child's dot to dot puzzle! The radiographers are kind to me, very aware of the pain, and they take their time. Not once do I feel rushed, or a nuisance.

And so the next day, Day One of the treatment, arrives and is to continue every weekday for the following month. The journey to and from the hospital becomes familiar. After my confinement for the past seven months, I feel liberated!

I discover that the treatment itself is painless to start with, although the discomfort of the 'zapping' makes itself known as the days go on. It takes longer to position me than it does to treat me, the radiographers reciting a litany of numbers and formulae which become familiar to me. I am aware that I take longer than the norm, as they gently take their time with my shoulder. I am treated with three separate bursts, in three sites, and the radiographers come in and out from behind their lead door to reposition and check each time.

Delays are inevitable. The new self-diagnosing equipment breaks down with regularity, and we spend some time waiting. It gives us the opportunity, we people in this 'exclusive club', to get to know each other. We meet each day, as old friends, and share our fears, our stories and our concerns for the future. Under the skin, we are all the same. We talk about wigs, hair loss, surgery, recovery and our discomforts in everyday life, unknown to others outside our club. We become almost intimate friends for a few days, and then we will go our separate ways, to continue our individual battles.

I am the only person in this little club to suffer from nausea and vomiting, as this side effect is apparently fairly uncommon among breast patients, I am told. The experienced kindly Clinic Sister who comes to see me on one memorably bad day says it is because I haven't had a chance to recover from the serious problems with chemotherapy, so have started from a very low point. She is very competent and reassuring, and once again, I feel well cared-for, and in safe hands.

I have made the decision that I wish to be followed up in this Centre, and on discussion with the Oncologist in my weekly review, I am told that whilst unusual, this should be possible. I am therefore reassured that should I ever (heaven forbid) need to be hospitalised in the future, I will already be in this hospital's 'system'. One of my reviews provides me with the opportunity of airing my questions with the Oncologist who is also Director of the Centre. He allows me so much time, and answers my questions candidly. Not all of the answers are reassuring, but I appreciate his honesty. The bottom line really is...............when you are finished here, go and enjoy your life, whilst being quietly aware of any possible changes occurring in your body. The future is unknown for everyone. Sound advice, I feel.

As the days of treatment roll on, my frequent physiotherapy sessions and the cortisone injection improve my lot considerably, and I can almost move my shoulder without too much pain. The radiotherapy sessions become quicker as I become more flexible. In addition, I have refined my dosage of anti-emetics, and am no longer very nauseous. It is a great relief!

Two thirds of the way through my twenty sessions I begin to experience a degree of discomfort in the radiation sites, and I frequently have shooting pains, but it is a small complaint, and I know it will soon be over. It is little more than painful sunburn, and I am told that the pains are nerve regeneration. That is an encouraging thought. I still experience some nausea too. Because of the discomfort in the treatment site, I tend to arrive at the hospital with two boobs in my jumper and leave with one of them in my bag! I appreciate my weekends off, which give me a chance to recover my strength, as the tiredness increases.

There are three radiotherapy machines in the department now, but each one of them frequently self-diagnoses a problem and shuts itself down, so there are still delays. It is disorientating to be in different rooms each day. Whilst the equipment is identical, the layout is at odds with what I'm used to. One room has light patterns on the ceiling for entertainment value. They use this room for the children. Again, a sobering thought.

And on the extremely positive side, my hair has started to grow! Of course, you would need a magnifying glass to see it. But the fuzz is there! As instructed, I have a baby's brush to use, but it won't be needed for a long time yet. My nails, also lost to chemotherapy, are now growing, although I later find that the second growth drops out too. Third time lucky perhaps! But my finger tips are far less painful now, although I cannot use my fingers well, and find this very frustrating. I have no feeling in the tips of them. I can't pick things up, turn pages, open things, or do buttons or zips up. I can't even scratch an itch!! And then, one by one, my painful toenails start to fall off!

At my last meeting with my Oncologist, I am advised that I won't have to visit a hospital again for two months. It is hard to believe that what people refer to as 'My Journey' is nearly over. It is eight months since this nightmare began. This final part has been made so easy for me because of the professionalism and kindness of the team here; from the gateman, who even remembers the day of my last treatment and wishes me luck in the future, through to the reception desk staff, the nursing and medical staff, and the radiographers. The Northern Centre for Cancer Care truly is a place of excellence. I feel sure that the excellence will continue even when the level of patients increases.

11th November at 11am

And so I approach my last treatment, ironically at 11am on the 11th of November. We herald it as our very own ceasefire!

For several days, I have been feeling very 'down' and tearful. It is strange and confusing to me, because I have yearned for this moment since the very beginning, nearly eight months ago. It is certainly not because I am loathe to leave the hospitals, and the various treatments. I can't wait to consign them to history. I can't wait to be in control of my own life again. I have dreamed of freedom for such a long time. I have been told that more people need counselling at this stage, than any of the preceding times. I am beginning to understand that, even if I can't understand why. I try to think it through, and reach the conclusion that for eight months, regardless of how terribly ill I have been, I have had to fight. I have had no choice but to face my enemy head on, and even in my weakest, most deadly state, I have had a purpose. My enemy was visible, palpable and an easy target for me.

Now I am left without knowing if I still have a fight on my hands; if I have won the war and not just the battle. I begin to realise I will never be free. I have to learn how to cope with the possibility of an invisible foe, and reach a balance of quiet vigilance, whilst loving and living my life.

Throughout my trials of the past months, I have so often said, 'I can't do this again!' Yet, with the wonderful help of those around me, I have bounced back each time, and gone on to do it again, and again, and again.

I shall take this philosophy with me into the unknown, with the certain knowledge that my life is worth fighting for. I haven't finished with it yet! I have so much more love to share.

CHRISTMAS LIGHTS

Words fall from the branches of her mind,
unmeasured.
They swirl and toss around the room,
and the elephant raises his head.

She sweeps them up,
but they fly free,
determined.

Denial cannot capture them,
although she does not speak them.
To hear them said
would make them real.

Rather, she would use the words
that heighten meaning;
escaping to a place
where thought cannot weave its complicated way,
and feeling is the only breath
within the secret space.

He weighs his words –
speckles of gold that settle in the scales of their unity;
precious dust of emotion.
He withholds them,
enriching them with rarity.

Treading his way carefully
over the sharpened stones of his mind,
the words he chooses
calm and still her,
questioning and analysing,
unpicking the tangled threads,
unravelling the knotted skeins,
sparkling,
like lights upon so many Christmas trees.

Chapter 8

JOURNEY'S END?

December

But of course, it isn't over; it will never be over. I am not even allowed a few weeks' grace.

A simple eye examination for new glasses gives me my first encounter with the 'freak-out', ironically just a few days before our long postponed holiday. I am told I have a naevus, a kind of mole, in my eye, and there is a 1% chance, in view of my recent problems, that it may be sinister, and I am told I must see an Ophthalmologist urgently. That measly 1% assumes such melodramatically high value in my head!

We have our long-awaited holiday, but it is filled with attempted urgent appointment-making, and worry. Once again, our General Practice takes the lead and makes arrangements for me, easing our pressures.

I daren't even enjoy my newly springing (well....a quarter of a centimetre!) hair, in case it's all taken away from me again. I return to the weepy, withdrawn stage, but try hard to be positive and practical.

Miraculously when the appointment arrives, I am told I have nothing to worry about. The Consultant is encouraging, and I only have to have the naevus measured every six months. To do this, I have to have the eyeball photographed. I come out of the consulting room and sit in the waiting room to await my turn with the medical photographer. I am crying, and in answer to a concerned question from a fellow patient, I reply that they are tears of relief. After all I have been through, I am so grateful to jump this hurdle. During the conversation with the medical photographer, I discover she too has survived cancer. I ask her if, after seven years of recovery, she still suffers from these 'freak-outs'.

The answer comes.............'all the time'!

≈≈≈≈≈

And life begins to return to normal at home...........well..........our version of normal!

I am under strict instructions to rest.

I try to pace myself, I really do. But the fates conspire, as I record in an email to a close friend:

This morning we got a phone call from our reliable builder who is 'fitting us in' ... a familiar phrase they use in their trade.

He also says he'll be here in ten minutes... yes, ten minutes, to fit the three new windows we had ordered a few days earlier ....den, kitchen and my study on the first floor.

That means a lot of moving around, especially in my study, and it also means yet more chips from the chip shop to ensure we do get something to eat today!

Having caused chaos in moving stuff around, they fit the downstairs rooms first, which gives me a bit of time to move my precious (to me) fossils and books to safety in my study.

Downstairs the new windows look beautiful: they have really done a great job.

And then they progress to upstairs...... and that means using a ladder.

They are nearly finished when an almighty crash occurs, and a man descends from the heavens and lands flat on his back in the garden in front of the kitchen window. I'm startled awake and I do my first aid exam of him, sort him out, and establish he's ok to move to sit in a chair.

The ladder (which was standing on the icy snow without anyone to hold it) is now bent double (as is the man) and there is a great big hole in the new kitchen window frame - the one they had finished just a short time earlier!

The man (who, we were then told, had also fallen from another roof two weeks ago) initially refused to go to hospital and limped around for ages, distracting his two accomplices and us until (two cups of tea and much chatter later) they all left. He had decided he would go for an x-ray in the hospital in his own town.

I guess someday we'll get a new kitchen window..........

Mind you - we were a tad worried because the ladder they used was an old (clearly broken) one of ours that was lying in the garden awaiting transport to the tip. Their own top quality, heavy duty, ladder was left sitting on top of their van...so Allan had to be around to pick up on any chat about liability etc - which ruined all his plans for the afternoon!

Just a typical day in our household during this awful year, but it has an added bonus of making me temporarily forget all about any lurking worries I might have.

2nd January 2009

The two months thus pass quickly, and suddenly it is today, the second day of a new year, Check-Up Day! We wonder if the events of this day will set a benchmark for the year. It is strange that these awesome events seem to surround memorable days: Easter Monday, our wedding anniversary, April Fools' Day, Allan's birthday. They are memorable enough in their own right without the added orchestration of interventions beyond our control.

As always, the build-up to it has been tense and all-consuming, but on the day, I am calm. My new white spikey hair and I are ready.

Amazingly, I have slept well for a change. This first follow-up appointment is in the old Regional Cancer Centre, not the new one because the outpatients' department is not quite ready. It is still nearly an hour's drive, but oh so much better than going locally and revisiting all those awful memories.

And in the end, it is easy. It is almost an anti-climax.

Allan and I sit in the vast hall of a waiting area. On this final occasion, I am allowed to mix with the other people there, and am not ushered into an isolated room. I can't help but look around and wonder about these people. But all of them seem so insulated and withdrawn. What are their stories? What stage have they reached? How far have they come? Which ones are wearing wigs? Tucked in the corner is a discreet little stall where you can buy headscarves and hats. I am grateful to no longer have any interest in this.

In the hushed stillness, our voices seem to echo.

A comfortable, but tense, wait and then my name is called. The Sister's face is familiar, and she remembers me from the Radiotherapy visits. Again, I feel I am among friends.

I am shown into a tiny examination room, and my Oncologist enters and asks me how I am! My answer is simple. I feel well, and 'me' for the first time in what seems a very long time.

A friend had warned that the examination would be quite thorough and "rough" but it certainly did not hurt in any way. The chat takes longer than the examination. Everything about this meeting seems so *normal,* so routine - this date that has assumed such a huge importance in my mind.

She draws a curtain to divide the room and then examines me. It is certainly not as uncomfortable as I had been expecting.

The thing I have dreaded is over. Two little words...'that's fine'.

I have been examined and-

I have passed my latest testing time!

She advises that I can improve my lot with a healthy diet and plenty of exercise. That makes me smile! With my sensitivities and allergies, if only it were that simple. The exercise bit doesn't pose a problem though. I have Sandy to ensure that! She also discusses breast reconstruction with me. I am not interested in pursuing this, but she advises me to keep an open mind in case I change it. But I have no intention of enduring anything else. I am content the way I am.

I make my next appointment at the desk, and skip out of the building a free woman!

It all seemed too easy, to be told quite simply, that all is well. There were no scans; no tests; no fanfare of trumpets; no shrieks of joy; no running along corridors sharing such vital information with all and sundry!

 Just an examination that says quite simply, all is well.

I am euphoric!

Allan and I share the huge relief. Our grins are as wide as the Tyne Bridge!

I don't have to go back for another three months. Three months of grace, when I can forget this, and begin my life again. And quietly, without fuss,

> ➢ my hair grows (the very first hair is a white one on my chin!);

- ➤ my fingernails repair themselves;

- ➤ I can do my own buttons up at last, and without pain in the fingertips;

- ➤ my toenails continue to drop off, exposing nice shiny new ones

- ➤ my radiation site begins to lose its blackness and soreness, mobility improving at the same time, although I have to be vigilant with exercises;

- ➤ my lumpy surgery site flattens making it more comfortable to wear my bra and my 'false leg';

- ➤ my taste buds, and therefore my appetite, are improving. I am able to eat a wider variety of food, although sweet food still tastes like poison and I still have a nasty taste;

I rarely need to use my Blue Badge, except when I recognise the need to save my energy. On those occasions, I am sometimes frowned at by other drivers who obviously think I'm swinging the lead. I no longer qualify for those little looks of sympathy, or blatant stares. Boy, does that feel good!

My energy and enthusiasm return, little by little, and my Survivor's Chart is littered with gold hearts!

Everyone is commenting the same thing.....' who would have thought it, just as little as two months ago, never mind the past year?'

Of course I over-do things, then have to succumb to resting, and then over-do things all over again! I can't help it. I have so much of my wonderful life to catch up with.

I sometimes become tearful and distressed when I tire easily, but rationality always kicks in, and I talk myself in and out of it (or someone does it for me!). When I am over-tired the fear creeps back, but mostly that door stays shut.

I am at last allowed to visit my dentist, something that is forbidden during treatment time because of susceptibility to infection, and danger of bleeding. As (my) luck would have it, I have had toothache for months, and by the time I go, I find I have to have root canal treatment and two crowns. I'm just grateful I am finally well enough to be able to go through with it.

I start to meet friends again, now I'm no longer so vulnerable. Not quite ready to drive any long distances yet, my first long-promised and exciting trip out is by train, to meet friends. It is cold, but I dance (in my fashion) on the beach like a liberated child. For months this outing has been dangled as the carrot for my improvement by these friends who have been cajoling and encouraging me via countless messages to my mobile phone, and online. It is one of the promises which kept my spirits up during the bad times. It may be a little too soon, as it tires me greatly, but it is SO worth it.

Returning on the train home, a bunch of Likely Lads sit down near me, off for their night on the 'Toon'. They cannot take their eyes off my baldy head. I no longer look like a Chemo-babe, but rather a 'Don't- Mess-With -Me -Babe!' It makes me smile.

Friends ask questions. "Has this experience changed me?"

Well on the lighter side....yes!

> I am a size or two thinner; my hair is surprisingly white, and shortly chic and curly, and I have been told by several people that I look healthier now than I have done for many years!

> I have encountered a whole new learning curve, discovering false breasts; stick on nipples; bras with secretive pockets; special camisoles with inserts to hide the missing cleavage.

> I have to be fitted for a smaller boob, because of the weight loss due to chemotherapy (you see, there's always a bright side!). It is lighter too, and more comfortable, and I feel and look completely 'normal' wearing it.

> I have to buy new clothes, when I not only have to consider my new size, but my new shape too since I can no longer wear some styles of tops and dresses.

> I also have to invest in a new pocketed swimsuit and a swimming prosthesis. This is a cause of great amusement! It looks and feels just like a transparent jellyfish. I wonder if it would be unwise to swim in the sea with it......I could experience unwelcome advances from male jellyfish! I have yet to try it out in the sea but I have worn it in a swimming pool. I think of it as my buoyancy aid. My husband tells me it is necessary to stop me swimming round in circles now that I am lopsided!

- ➢ I have been bolstered up by 'keep your hair on' and 'I'll wear my single breasted suit to match you, dear' jokes. A year on they, and many more, are still used continually.

- ➢ One of my Christmas presents from my daughter was lash-lengthening mascara! *(my eyebrows and lashes have now returned).*

It's a good thing I do have a sense of humour! In fact, my original title for this book was 'One Tassel and a Jellyfish', but I was persuaded that it might be misinterpreted, and so I changed it!

I have been told many times, by many people, how well I have taken all of this; how my sense of humour has amazed them; how they could not have coped. But when fate delivers a blow such as this, what choice do you have if you want to live?

As I pass the first anniversary of the day my world turned upside down, I cannot believe how far I have come, for

- ➢ I am singing again, and performing in concerts.

- ➢ I have started back at school, albeit on a very limited basis.

- ➢ I have registered to do the 'Race for Life' in aid of Cancer Research (although it must be said I intend to walk!). And any surplus from the sale of this book will benefit that charity.

- ➢ I am out and about again, with no thought of 'being careful' all the time.

- ➢ I am gardening (yes, Headstrong ladies..........with gloves and sunscreen!).

- ➢ Almost as a postscript to this book I can add that 54 weeks after discovering the egg, I have now had my first haircut!

I feel I have my life back, and it is good. My blessings multiply.

On the downside ...I'm also capable of ironing again!!

It has not been an easy year, to say the least. But I have been carried through it all; supported, chivvied and organised; and loved, always loved. I have done none of it on my own. The pain has been mine, but I have never once borne it alone.

My husband, daughter, daughter-in-law, son and ma-in-law supported me beyond measure, bearing the load between them. Not once have they let me down, and I have watched the younger generation blossom and mature. I have become the child, and they the parents. There will never be enough words to tell them all how much I appreciate them. Sadly Mum died recently, but I was proud to be able to give the eulogy at her funeral.

My friends have been constantly 'by my side', mostly by letters, phone-calls, texts and emails, since they were rarely allowed near me, but never once leaving me alone or lonely. They have been amazing with their kindness:

- ➢ one of my dearest friends, whose day always begins by talking to me 'on line';

- ➢ texts which arrive several times a day from another special friend who will not allow me to sink into self-pity;

- ➢ special non-allergy cakes made by another special friend for the rare occasions I was able to eat;

- ➢ books given for the equally rare times I was able to read;

- ➢ exquisite hand-made cards in abundance from another friend;

- ➢ 'annoying' comic cards and notes from a friend who wrote without fail every few days with snippets of nonsense that never failed to make me smile;

- ➢ vases never empty of flowers;

- ➢ notes of encouragement and inspiration, and 'pull-yourself-together-girl' advice;

- ➢ practical gifts of pens and books to write in, and socks to keep me warm;

- ➢ amusing gifts to make me smile.

- ➢ 'baby-sitters' for the times Allan had to leave me to be with his Mum;

➢ one of my closest friends who would lie on the bed with me, holding my hand and stroking my head, running for the vomit bowl, staying silent or talking whenever the mood dictated.

➢ friends who never gave up phoning, even though most of the time I was too ill or too tired to talk to them;

➢ a cleric client of Allan's (and now a good friend to us both) who was happy just to sit quietly or to natter if I felt like it, as well as, along with many others, to brighten our house with flowers

➢ sensible, practical advice from those who had been on this journey before me.

How would I have survived without them?

They have loved me through it all, providing the comfort of words I so desperately need. It is impossible to underestimate the solace this has brought me. People I considered as distant friends have become close. I have been so privileged to experience the generosity of the human spirit.

I have been told that the world will look different to me now- the grass greener, trees and flowers more beautiful, colours richer. But the world has always been that way to me. I have always appreciated it, as I have always appreciated my life and my loves.

My childhood friend in Australia, and my first young love, whom we had visited a few months before this happened to me, wrote a poem to match a photograph he has also sent to me. It is of a tree, ravaged by fire and storms, and seemingly dead or dying. But out of its blackened, burned and damaged trunk, this springtime it bravely displayed new healthy leaves, in wonderful rich colour. My friend has named it his Eucalyptus Sue!

If this experience has changed me at all, it is in the strengthening confirmation of something I have always lived by: we must make the best of what we have been given; lose no time in regret; accept the things we cannot change; fight for those things we can. And always, always, live life to the full.

I wrote the following poem a few years ago.

I can think of no more meaningful words with which to conclude this latest chapter of my life:

ETERNAL SPRING

Autumn colours blaze
in splendid loveliness
around me.
Seasons mingle in my head;
leaves turn catkin yellow,
tulip red,
and float like cherry blossom
down to mellow earth
confusing me.

Mists weave their way
like early morning dew.
Golden tendrils drape
from shrubbery and vine,
bewitching me.
My future memories
plant their seeds anew,
enticingly.

I will not bow to seasons,
conform to expectations
constricting me.
No Autumn in my life,
but sweet and beautiful eternal Spring.

Chapter 9

REFLECTIONS

If it is not too much of a self indulgence, I would like to pass on to you a little of what I have learned, not just in this past year, but throughout my eventful life, including my short nursing career which was abruptly brought to a halt after suffering my first 'slipped' disc.

Members of the Medical Profession, however talented, are not gods. They have human failings, as do we all. They get tired, stressed, over-worked, and anxious for their patients, at the same time as progressing their own careers. But one way or another, they learn from each of their patients, and move on to the next one.

We have just the one body (obvious, but true!), and it is our own responsibility, not theirs. *We* have to ask the questions of them, and discuss our problems and worries.

If necessary, when you visit a health professional, take a list of your questions and take someone with you who will help you remember all the answers you are given.

And if they have not explained things to your satisfaction, ask repeatedly, and don't leave until you have an answer!! It is up to you to share your concerns with them. They have no idea what you are thinking or feeling unless you tell them. They cannot make guesses.

And if you are still not happy, seek a second opinion. It is your right. Don't just accept what they are doing to you, or what they tell you. Question everything! You really don't have to put your precious life in the hands of just one person. The responsibility is too great for a fallible fellow human being, and to do so is too much of a risk for you.

The decision not to name everyone I encountered on this journey was taken to prevent concern for patients who may be attending the same local hospital.

Remember EVERYONE IS DIFFERENT!

Chapter 10

EUCALYPTUS SUE

Four months prior to the discovery of my "duck egg", Allan and I had been in Queensland, Australia where I was able to meet my very first 'boy friend' Mick Fisher from long, long, ago!

We had miraculously re-discovered each other a few years earlier and the visit was especially to see Mick (now known as Mike - but he will always be Mick to me!) again, and meet his wonderful wife Pam. For those of you who might wonder how such re-unions fare, in our case we all got on really well and had a wonderful time together!

Having maintained regular contact with me throughout my illness, as I was emerging from the nightmare of the past year, Mick sent me a photograph of "his" gum tree and with it, the following words – which I treasure:

The gum tree stands on the edge of the bush
And as long as I've lived here, I pass it each day
It seems that all it would take is one decent push
And it would fall, and if not, at least sway

Mutilated many years ago by a sudden storm
And at least four bush fires that occur down-under
It endures, ravaged and savaged and disfigured in form
A symbol of defiance, always a source of wonder

The base of its trunk is exposed to termites and fire
Yet this spring it bravely displayed new leaves of green
Its meagre branches thrust them higher and higher
As a symbol of resilience and endurance, it has to be seen

It clings to life with much courage and defiance
And the richness of its foliage, such a wonderful hue
It defies what should have been, according to science
So I have named this tree my
"Eucalyptus Sue"

The Author:

Sue Percival was born and educated in North London, but spent her childhood in the wilds of Hampshire: '*my mother was of gypsy heritage, and I soon developed a strong affinity for the countryside and nature; from my father came a lifelong zeal for words and music.*'

She moved to the North East shortly after marrying and began writing poetry and prose seriously in 2002. Sue currently enjoys the opportunity to share her passion for the written word with primary school children in the region, and her poetry has been appreciated in several countries.

This journal is an instinctive and vital account of a year spent within the clutches of breast cancer and the British medical system.

Further titles by Sue include:

The Horizon Of My Mind

Morning Meeting

And for children:

No Tail

Snuffly

Details of these can be found at

www.anchorage-publications.co.uk